Laser Techniques in Ophthalmology

Laser Techniques in Ophthalmology

A Guide to YAG and Photothermal Laser Treatments in Clinic

Anita Prasad, MBBS, FRCOphth
Royal Gwent Hospital, Aneurin Bevan University Health Board

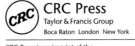

CRC Press
Taylor & Francis Group
Boca Raton London New York

CRC Press is an imprint of the
Taylor & Francis Group, an **informa** business

First edition published 2022
by CRC Press
6000 Broken Sound Parkway NW, Suite 300, Boca Raton, FL 33487-2742

and by CRC Press
2 Park Square, Milton Park, Abingdon, Oxon, OX14 4RN

© 2022 Taylor & Francis Group, LLC

CRC Press is an imprint of Taylor & Francis Group, LLC

Library of Congress Cataloging-in-Publication Data
Names: Prasad, Anita G., 1978– author.
Title: Laser techniques in ophthalmology: a guide to YAG and photothermal
laser treatments in clinic/by Anita Prasad.
Description: First edition. | Boca Raton, FL: CRC Press, 2022. |
Includes bibliographical references and index. |
Summary: "This is a practical guide to using lasers in the eye clinic and includes all commonly performed lasers for a range of ocular conditions. It standardizes laser procedures and serves as a reference guide for ophthalmic trainees learning the technique that can be transferred to their clinical practice"– Provided by publisher.
Identifiers: LCCN 2021062227 (print) | LCCN 2021062228 (ebook) |
ISBN 9780367700324 (hardback) | ISBN 9780367700317 (paperback) | ISBN 9781003144304 (ebook)
Subjects: MESH: Eye Diseases–surgery | Laser Therapy–methods |
Lasers, Solid-State–therapeutic use | Handbook
Classification: LCC RE80 (print) | LCC RE80 (ebook) |
NLM WW 39 | DDC 617.7/1–dc23/eng/20220113
LC record available at https://lccn.loc.gov/2021062227
LC ebook record available at https://lccn.loc.gov/2021062228

ISBN: 9780367700324 (hbk)
ISBN: 9780367700317 (pbk)
ISBN: 9781003144304 (ebk)

DOI: 10.1201/9781003144304

Typeset in Palatino
by Newgen Publishing UK

Printed in the UK by Severn, Gloucester on responsibly sourced paper

*To my husband, Ajay, and children, Aditya and Tapasya, my pride and joy,
for inspiring me to excel in everything I do.*

To my parents for encouraging me to believe in myself.

To my family and friends for being there for me.

*To my teachers and mentors, who have taught me over the years, and trainees,
who have been a source of inspiration, learning, and constant evolution.*

Table of Contents

Acknowledgements

Writing this book has been a rewarding and fulfilling experience. **I hope to bring a trainer's perspective, giving essential laser training some structure, based on knowledge and clinical experience.**

The book concentrates on common laser techniques in the eye clinic, bringing clarity on treatment concepts, techniques, and plans, developing good clinical practice and skill sets, with an easy to understand, user-friendly approach, using multiple digitally enhanced illustrations, for ready reference in the laser clinic.

A big thanks to Amy, Tom, and Mike from medical illustration, for their help and advice in collating images for the book.

To the trainees who jogged my memory, and proofread the book in its early stages with encouraging feedback. Thank you, Luke, Francis, Alex, James, Connor, Sejal, Shoaib, and Ellie. I hope you learnt as much from me as I have from teaching you.

Thanks to Gwyn and Patrick for their initial input and encouragement, and to Shivangi, Himani, and everyone on the publishing team. I could not have done this without your help.

Trainee Feedback

I am not aware of any existing book that approaches this subject in this way. I think ophthalmic trainees nationally and internationally would find appeal in a book that provides a structured theoretical grounding in the subject with a practical approach to using ophthalmic lasers. The use of illustrations is vital for teaching this subject and the approach used by annotating these images in this book is ideal for demonstrating techniques.

LP

The pictures are good, in particular I like the treatment plan ones with areas you might deliver lasers. I would have felt a lot more confident having read this before doing my own cases. I think the format with boxes is good with good snippets of information.

JP

About the Author

Anita Prasad is an ophthalmologist with an interest in medical retina, with over 25 years of experience, and a laser lead and trainer at ABUHB Trust for over 20 years. **It has given her a unique insight and approach into an area that is not well taught, using digitally** **enhanced images to highlight learning points and simplify techniques, making it easy for learners to get started with lasers.** Outside of medical work, Anita is an artist, dabbling in oils and acrylics, and enjoys reading, cooking, and community work.

Glossary

Absorb: To transform radiant energy into a different form, usually with a resultant rise in temperature

Amplification: Growth of the radiation field in the resonator cavity from multiple reflections between the cavity mirrors

Amplitude: The maximum value of electromagnetic wave height

Bandwidth: The width of the optical spectrum of light, expressed in wavelength units (m) or frequency units (Hz)

Brightness: The luminous power of a light beam

Coherence: Waves that are synchronized, with phase difference between their oscillations remaining constant as they propagate. This allows laser light to be concentrated into small spots, or ultra-small pulses

Collimation: Process by which divergent rays (natural light) are converted to parallel rays

CNV: Choridal neovascular membrane

CW mode: Continuous emission of electromagnetic wave of constant frequency or wavelength and amplitude, at constant power

Depth of field: The working range of the beam, based on wavelength and laser focusing mechanisms

Energy: Measurement of laser light to induce change (heating / cutting), measured in watts. Energy is inversely proportional to wavelength.

Excited state: State of higher energy of an atom or molecule

Flashlamp: Source of powerful light used to excite stimulated emission in a solid-state laser

Flux: The radiant or luminous power of a light beam

Fluence: All laser irradiance = laser irradiance + any backscattered irradiance.

Frequency: Number of light waves / complete vibrations in a fixed period of time. Frequency is inversely proportional to the wavelength of light

IOL: Intraocular lens

Irradiance: Laser power per unit area = watts / cm^2. It is a measure of how strongly laser works on a given tissue

Gain: The increase in energy through amplification

Gain medium: The lasing medium that provides the atoms / molecules for stimulated emission and coherent amplification

Ground state: The state of lowest stable energy level in an atom or molecule

Heat sink: Substance or device used to absorb or dissipate unwanted heat

Hertz (Hz): Measurement of frequency of light (cycles / second)

Intensity: Magnitude of radiant energy / light per unit time or area

Joules: Measurement of laser energy in time – watts / second, for pulsed laser

Lifetime: Time taken for an excited atom to spontaneously decay back to ground state or a lower energy state

Luminance: The flux / unit area

Monochromatic: Light consisting of single wavelength of light

Nanometre: Unit of length = 1 billionth of a meter, used to measure wavelength

OHT: ocular hypertension

Optical density: Protection factor of eyewear filter used with lasers. Each unit of OD represents ×10 increase in eye protection

Optical fibre: Light or laser transmitting optical material for great distances

Optical pump: Exciting a lasing material using light as the external source

PCO: Posterior capsular opacification

Photon: Smallest packet of light energy. Energy is directly proportional to the frequency of light

Population inversion: State when the atoms in the excited state exceed atoms in the ground state; forms the basis for stimulated emission

Power: Energy / unit time measured in watts. Power is constant in CW laser or variable in a pulsed laser

Power density: Laser power / surface area (spot size) on which it works. Increasing power or decreasing spot size will increase power density. Excessive power density can rupture Bruch's membrane and cause choroidal neovascularisation.

POAG: Primary Open angle glaucoma

Pulsed mode: Light emitted in short bursts or pulses of highly concentrated energy. Energy of laser in pulsed mode is much greater than CW lasers

Q-switch: Shutter device that allows laser energy to be released in small pulses. Energy is only released when it reaches a higher power

Radiance: A measure of how strong a laser is

Raman effect: When a wavelength of light can be changed by molecular scattering

Refractive Index: Property of a medium that determines how light propagates through it. RI of vacuum is 1 and of water is 1.33 (This means that light travels 1.33 times more slowly in water than vacuum). RI determines how light bends when passing through a medium. RI of lens – 1.386, vitreous – 1.336, RI of silicon oil > RI of vitreous

Resonator: The optical cavity with mirrors on each end that amplifies the stimulated emission, generating a laser beam

Spontaneous emission: Emission of a photon of light by spontaneous decay of an excited atom

Stimulated emission: External source of energy / photon that stimulates atoms to get excited and achieve population inversion; forms the basis of laser light generation

Wavelength: The distance an EM wave travels during 1 cycle of oscillation. Property of light that determines its colour, measured in nanometres. Monochromatic light has a single wavelength, while polychromatic light is multi-coloured. Wavelength determines how effectively light penetrates ocular media and how well it is absorbed by the target tissue

Introduction

LASER is an acronym for **L**ight **A**mplification by **S**timulated **E**mission of **R**adiation. To lase is to absorb energy in one form and emit a new more useful form of energy.

Lasers were first conceptualized by Albert Einstein (1917). The first prototype photothermal laser was built by Theodore Maiman (1960), and they have since become essential tools in ophthalmic practice. Recent technological advances and new concepts have renewed interest in the topic.

Lasers can be generated in a spectrum of wavelengths (short UV to long IR) with a multitude of applications including electronics, information technology, science, medicine, entertainment, military, industry, and law enforcement. Modern fibre-optic communication technology such as the Internet uses lasers.

haemorrhages. Surgical lasers can cut, coagulate, and remove tissues, with minimal, no-touch techniques, improving outcomes. **New concepts and advances have improved laser safety and delivery** including eye-tracking feature, subthreshold, shorter pulse and multispot lasers.

Lasers have branched into diagnostic realms, including the laser-based microscopic technique for early diagnosis of ocular (ARMD, glaucoma) and neurodegenerative conditions like Alzheimer's disease. Laser technology is used in investigative techniques such as laser interferometry, spectroscopy, microperimetry mapping of macula, confocal scanning laser ophthalmoscope (CSLO), optical coherence tomography (OCT and OCT-A), and laser retinal Doppler flowmetry.

0.1 LASERS IN OPHTHALMOLOGY (DIAGNOSTIC AND THERAPEUTIC)

Lasers can reshape corneas to improve focus, improve IOP in glaucoma and cauterize

Anatomical site	Laser procedure	Type of laser
Ocular adnexa	Removal of lid lesions, blepharoplasty, removal of wrinkles, capillary haemangioma, and port-wine stain, DCR	CO_2 laser
Cornea (keratorefractive surgery)	PRK (photorefractive keratectomy), laser in-situ keratomeleusis (LASIK), laser subepithelial keratectomy (LASEK), phototherapeutic keratectomy (PTK), laser for corneal neovascularization	Excimer laser
Sclera	Laser scleroplasty, laser suture lysis (post trabeculectomy)	Holmium YAG Argon/PASCAL
Iris	Peripheral iridotomy (PI), laser iridoplasty, laser pupilloplasty	Nd-YAG laser, Argon/PASCAL
Angle	Selective laser trabeculoplasty (SLT), PASCAL SLT	Nd-YAG laser
Ciliary Body	Cyclophotocoagulation (CPC) scleral/pupillary/endoscopic	Diode, Nd-YAG
Lens	Cataract surgery (incision, capsulorhexis, nuclear photo-fragmentation) – FLACS – femtolaser assisted cataract surgery, PCO	Femtolaser Nd-YAG laser
Vitreous	Viterolysis	Nd-YAG laser
Posterior Segment	PRP, FLT, Sectoral PRP, retinopexy, laser for ARMD, IO tumours, and other vasculopathies	Argon, PASCAL, Diode

DOI: 10.1201/9781003144304-1

1

Other Medical Applications of Lasers	
Speciality lasers	**Uses**
Dermatology CO_2 (10600 nm), Pulsed dye (585–595 nm), Nd-YAG (1064 nm), Ho-YAG (2090 nm), Er-YAG (2940 nm), ruby laser (694 nm), alexandrite (755 nm), HeNe laser, diode laser	Cosmetic surgery – removal of tattoo, birthmarks, sunspots, stretchmarks, scars, wrinkles, hair removal, skin resurfacing and rejuvenation, management of burns, surgical scars, scar contractures, lipolysis, body contouring, removal of freckles, naevi, keratosis, viral warts, vascular/pigmented congenital lesions, acne, cellulite, and striae reduction.
Urology – YAG, thallium fibre laser	Renal stones – lithotripsy, BPH.
Rheumatology, gynaecology, ENT, surgery – CO_2, Er-YAG, HeNe, GaAs laser	Soft tissue surgery, laser scalpel.
Dentistry – HeNe, GaAs, diode, mid-IR lasers	Teeth whitening, endodontic, and periodontic procedures.
Neurosurgery – CO_2, Nd-YAG, argon	Precise removal of brain and spinal cord tumours.
Orthopaedic – diode laser	Cartilage resurfacing and reshaping.
Oncology – dye, metal vapour **laser laser** induced interstitial thermotherapy (LITT)	Superficial skin cancers (BCC, SCC), endothelial – penile, vulval, vaginal, cervical, early non-small cell lung cancer.
Cardiothoracic – argon laser, Nd-YAG laser, CO_2 laser	Coronary artery disease, ventricular and supraventricular arrhythmias, hypertrophic cardiomyopathy, laser thrombolysis, trans-myocardial laser revascularization.

THERAPEUTIC ROLE OF LASERS IN OPHTHALMOLOGY

Section 1 Basic Principles of Laser

This section deals with basic laser principles and their applications in the eye clinic. It gives an overview and understanding of laser physics, delivery, safety, and pathophysiology for safe laser treatment.

1.1 LASER PHYSICS

Laser light differs from ordinary light, with special properties, making it clinically useful.

1.1.1 Properties of Laser Light

1. **Coherent** – all wavelengths are in phase, to accurately focus the beam, allowing precise experiments and measurements.

   - **Coherence allows laser light to be manipulated longitudinally to create short pulses or transversely to get small spots.**

2. **Polarized** – all wavelengths vibrate in one plane.

3. **Monochromatic** – light of single wavelength or frequency or colour. Monochromaticity reduces chromatic aberration and allows selective tissue targeting, based on the tissue absorption spectrum.

   - Ordinary light (natural or artificial) is multicoloured, with a range of visible and invisible (ultraviolet and infrared) wavelengths. A fluorescent lamp has a narrow spectral emission, coloured LED (light emitting diodes) have narrower bandwidth, and He-Ne laser bandwidth is extremely narrow at 632.8 nm (red).

   - **Monochromaticity is not essential; some lasers emit a range of wavelengths.**

4. **Collimated – all waves are unidirectional, parallel over long distances and remain intense and focused** (ordinary light diverges and becomes less bright). **Collimation allows precise focus without losing beam intensity.**

Lasers can be manipulated to make them useful in practice:

- **Ability to be concentrated in short intervals,** generating intense pulses.

- **Ability to produce non-linear effects** – non-linear absorption, refraction, decrease transmission, frequency doubling, Raman effect, frequency amplification, mode locking, and Q-switching.

1.1.2 Understanding Laser Physics

Molecules are made up of atoms, with a central positively charged nucleus (protons and neutrons), orbited by negatively charged electrons.
   Ground state (non-excited state) is the lowest possible energy state of an atom. Electrons in ground state absorb energy and rise to an **excited state** (higher orbit).

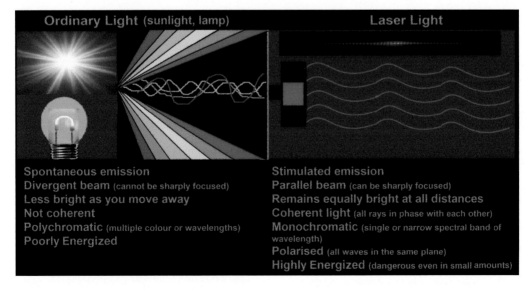

Figure 1.1 Ordinary light vs laser light.

DOI: 10.1201/9781003144304-2

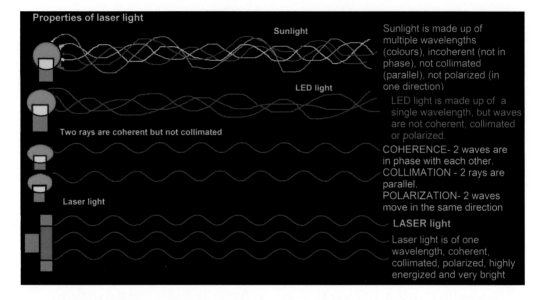

Figure 1.2 Properties of laser light.

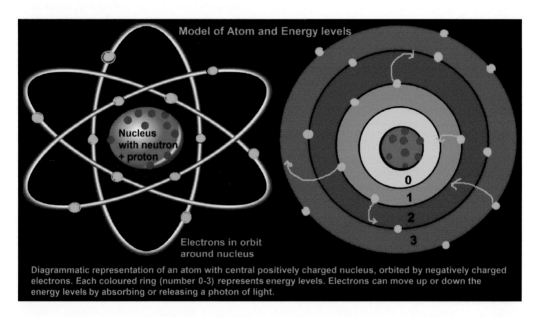

Figure 1.3 Atom and energy levels.

- **Light is an electromagnetic wave, emitting radiant energy in tiny packets called photons or quanta.**

- **E = hv** (E is energy in joules, h is frequency of light in hertz, and v is Planck's constant = 6.626×10^{-34} joules times second).

- Each photon has a characteristic frequency or wavelength.

- The **energy of a photon depends on its frequency or wavelength.**

- Wavelength is inversely related to frequency. High frequency = short wavelength, and vice versa. Wavelength (λ) is measured in nanometres.

- One **wavelength** is the distance between 2 successive wave crests or troughs.

- **Frequency** is the number of waves per second, measured in hertz. Higher frequency light has more waves/second (shorter wavelength).

- Energy is directly proportional to frequency – higher frequency has higher energy and a shorter wavelength.

- The blue and UV end of the spectrum has more energy than the red or IR end of the spectrum.

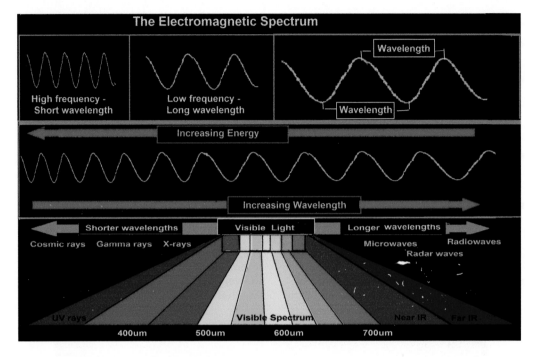

Figure 1.4 The electromagnetic spectrum.

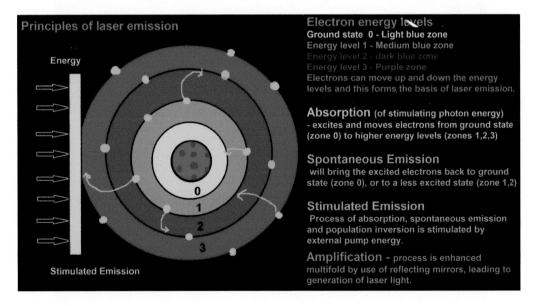

Figure 1.5 Principles of laser emission.

1.1.3 How Does an Atom in the Ground State Move to an Excited State?

- Normally, atoms in a medium are in a stable, low-energy ground state. **When a photon** of light stimulates it, electrons absorb the photon energy and move up to an excited, higher energy state – **absorption**.

- Electrons do not stay excited forever. They decay spontaneously by releasing energy and move down to a lower level of energy or back to the ground state.

- The decay time is called **lifetime.**

- Decay to a lower orbit releases a photon (energy) – **spontaneous emission.**

- The energy of an emitted photon is the difference between the stimulating energy and end energy (same as the stimulating energy if decay is to ground level or lower if decay is to a less excited level).

- **The emitted photon has the same phase, direction, and wavelength as the stimulating photon.**

- **So, transition of electrons up or down the orbit is accompanied by absorption or emission of a replica photon.**

1.1.4 Stimulated Emission

- Absorption excites atoms. If more photons strike the atom, it stimulates more and more electrons at ground state to get excited or already excited atoms to reach higher levels of energy. Eventually, a point is reached where the number of excited electrons is greater than electrons in ground state – **population inversion.**

- Population inversion leads to spontaneous emission of higher energy photons, which stimulates more electrons – **stimulated emission.**

- If this process is repeated multiple times, it generates an extremely high level of energy – **light amplification.**

- The newly emitted photons have the same frequency and direction as the stimulating photons. **Stimulated emission is effectively a process of cloning photons, amplifying light, and forms the core principle of laser action.**

The photons generated are monochromatic, collimated, coherent, highly energized, and very bright. These are all features of laser light.

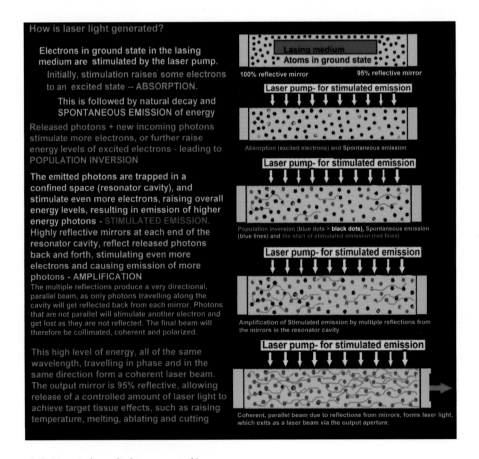

Figure 1.6 How is laser light generated?

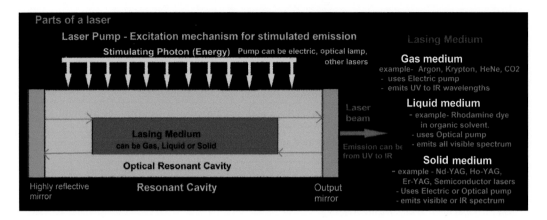

Figure 1.7 Parts of a laser.

1.1.5 Parts of a Laser

A laser comprises a pump, lasing medium, and resonator cavity.

- A **laser pump is the external energy source** that excites the lasing medium and triggers stimulated emission.

- **Gain/lasing medium** (provides atoms for stimulated emission)

- **Optical resonator** – cavity around the lasing medium with mirrors to amplify stimulated emission and an aperture to allow release of a laser beam for clinical effect.

Laser pump – External energy to excite atoms and start process of stimulated emission.	
Pumping can be by	**Variety of laser pumps used**
• Continuous discharge lamp for CW laser	• Optical pump – flashlamp, arc lamps, light from another laser (diode).
• Intermittent flashlamp for intermittent pulses.	• Chemical reactions
	• Explosive devices
	• Electric currents in semiconductors.
	• Pulse duration varies from CW to femtoseconds.
	• A laser can fire a single shot or repetitive bursts of pulses.

Laser or gain medium – Determines laser properties and emitted wavelength.

Provides atoms, electrons, or ions to be excited by the pump.

Gas lasers – Gas enclosed in a tube and pumped by electrical discharge. Three types:

	Atomic lasers	**Ionic lasers**	**Molecular lasers**
Example	Helium-neon	Argon, krypton	CO_2 laser
Pump	Electric	Electric	Electric, radio waves
Lasing medium	Neon atoms	Argon, krypton ion	CO_2 molecule (10–15% CO_2 gas)
Role of other molecules	Helium carries electric charge to neon atom		Nitrogen is transport gas Helium is heat sink gas
Wavelength emitted	633 nm, used in optical research labs	315–529 nm 458, 488, 514 nm	10600 nm – thermal IR in cutting, welding, used in dermatology

Liquids lasers – Active medium is an organic dye (rhodamine), dissolved in a liquid solvent (ethanol or ethylene glycol), in a glass chamber, pumped by another laser; emits across entire EM spectrum.

Free Electron Lasers (FEL) – Active medium is an electron beam from a particle accelerator. Generates tuneable wavelengths in widest frequency range of any laser.

Excimer lasers – excited diatomic molecule (excited dimer) – electrical pumping forms an unstable diatomic molecule (from union of 2 rare gases or a rare gas with a halogen). UV emission occurs when unstable diatom dissociates back to the constituent atoms. Examples: *argon fluoride – 193 nm, krypton chloride – 222 nm, krypton fluoride – 248 nm, xenon chloride*

Metal-vapor lasers – hybrids lasers (features of atomic and ionic lasers). Examples: helium-cadmium laser, helium-copper, helium-gold lasers.

Chemical lasers – two highly reactive gases form a molecule which becomes the lasing medium. Emit IR spectrum (2700 nm–3800 nm). Example: hydrogen fluoride (HF).

Solids state lasers – use cylindrical crystal (YAG, sapphire) or glass rod that has been doped with the active lasing medium. The crystal is used for its mechanical, thermal, and optical properties.

- **The dopant or lasing medium is a 1% impurity such as chromium, erbium, neodymium, titanium, holmium, and ytterbium ions added to the crystal.**

- **Normally, solid state lasers emit in the infrared spectrum but can be made to emit a wide range of wavelengths by using a variety of crystals and harmonic generation or frequency doubling.**

- *Example: Nd-YAG emits 1064 nm (IR), but can be frequency-doubled 532 nm PASCAL (green, visible), tripled – 355 nm, and quadrupled – 266 nm (UV) rays, by using KTP crystal.*

- **They are pumped by a flashlamp or light from another laser.** *A flashlamp is not the most effective as 70% is wasted as heat in the crystal, requiring cooling.*

- **A laser-generating higher frequency-monochromatic light is a better pump (diode laser).**

- A CW solid laser causes tissue heating (IR emissions), and is **best operated in a pulsed mode, using Q-switch or mode lock to generate ultra-short pulses.**

Dopant	Examples of laser	Wavelength generated
Neodymium	Nd – yttrium aluminium garnet (YAG) Nd – yttrium orthovandate (Nd-YVO4) Nd – yttrium lithium fluoride (Nd-YLF)	Near IR – 1064 nm, can be made to emit other wavelengths (tuneable)
Titanium	Ti – sapphire laser	IR, highly tuneable
Holmium	Ho – YAG laser	Far IR – 2097 nm
Chromium	Cr – sapphire laser (ruby laser)	Near IR spectrum

The resonator cavity – optical cavity around the laser medium with highly reflective mirrors at each end, to reflect photons multiple times, cause amplification, and improve laser efficiency.

- **Amplification and directionality of beam** – multiple reflections increase energy exponentially; only parallel beams get reflected.

- **Use of other optical devices** – spinning mirrors, modulators, absorbers, filters, and crystals, placed in the cavity to alter laser wavelength or pulses' duration.

- **Provides means of controlling laser usage** – output mirror is 95% reflective, allowing controlled release of laser for tissue effect.

1.2 PARAMETERS OF LASER LIGHT – DETERMINES ITS TISSUE BIOLOGICAL EFFECTS

Laser is defined by three parameters: wavelength, power, and mode.

1.2.1 Laser Wavelength

Spectrum of wavelengths (measured in nanometres and micrometres) – Determined by the lasing medium and defines tissue penetration, allowing optimal wavelength selection for specific tissue targets.

Spectrum		Laser type	Wavelength	
Far IR **Mid IR** **Near IR**		CO_2 laser Er-YAG Ho-YAG Nd-YAG Diode	10,600 nm 2940 nm 2120 nm 1064 nm 810 nm	Infrared wavelengths cause thermal effects on tissues
Visible spectrum **400 nm–750 nm**		Diode laser Ruby laser Krypton HeNe laser HeNe laser Dye laser PASCAL laser Argon laser	680 nm 694 nm – red 647 nm – red 632 nm – red–orange 543 nm – green 570–630 nm – yellow 532 nm – green 514 nm – green 488 nm – blue	Visible range wavelengths cause photochemical reactions
Ultraviolet		Excimer laser XeF – xenon fluoride XeCl – xenon chloride Nd-YAG solid laser Nd-YLF solid laser KrF – krypton fluoride ArF – argon fluoride	351 nm 308 nm 266 nm (freq quad) 263 nm (freq quad) 248 nm 193 nm	Shorter wavelengths have higher energy UV lasers energy > IR lasers energy

Common Lasers Used in Ophthalmology

	IR lasers	Visible lasers	UV lasers
	High wavelength lower energy	**Red, yellow, and green lasers**	**Shorter wavelength higher energy**
Laser type and wavelength and pulse duration	**CO_2** – 9.2–10.8 μm, **CW or ms pulsed** **Er-YAG** – 2.94 μm, **100–250 ns pulsed** **Ho-YAG** – 2.1 μm, **100–250ns pulsed** **Nd-YAG** – 1064 nm, **100ps – CW** **Nd-YLF** – 1053 nm, **100ps –CW** **Ti-Sapph** – 700–1000 nm, **60fs – 10ps pulsed** **Diode** – 635–1550 nm, **1ns – CW** **Alexandrite** – 720–800 nm, **50 ns–100 μs**	**Ruby laser**- 694 nm, **1–250 μs** **Krypton** – 531, 568, 647 nm, **CW or ms pulsed** **HeNe** – 633 nm, **CW** **PASCAL** – 532 nm (freq doubled Nd-YAG), **ms pulsed** Nd-YLF (freq-doubled) – 532 nm **Argon** – 488 and 514 nm, **CW or ms pulsed. Argon blue (488 nm) no longer used due to risk of macular burn**	**ArF Excimer laser** – 193 nm, **3–20 ns pulsed** KrCl (222 nm), KrF (248 nm), XeBr (282 nm), XeCl (308 nm), XeF (351 nm) **Gas lasers** – second harmonic bands of ionic and metal vapour lasers such as argon – 363–275 nm krypton – 356, 350, 337 nm He-Cd laser – 325 nm gold (Au) laser – 312 nm. *These are examples of visible lasers emitting in UV range by using frequency doubling.*
Laser effect	Absorbed by tissues with high water content, useful for surgical and thermal effects. IR lasers generate heat used in cutting and welding. **Thermal, mechanical, photochemical**	Red, green, and yellow lasers are well absorbed by the RPE, making them ideal for **thermal photocoagulation. Thermal Imaging** (HeNe) laser	High energy breaks molecular bonds and ionizes tissues, without thermal effects. Allows precise tissue sculpting and useful in corneal remodelling and cataract surgery – **photoablation**

1.2.2 Tuneable Lasers

Wavelength output of lasers depends on the lasing material, its refractive index (RI), length, and optical features of the resonator cavity (that alter laser oscillations), wavelength of laser pump, and substances or crystals added, to alter properties of the lasing material.

- **Frequency doubling** – alters long IR wavelengths into short visible and UV ranges;

- **Raman scattering** converts shorter wavelengths into longer wavelengths (far IR).

Lasers can be made to emit variable wavelengths by altering the optical cavity, lasing material, pumping mechanism, or the addition of frequency-changing crystals.

Common non-linear crystals used are KTP (Potassium titanyl phosphate), KDP (potassium dihydrogen phosphate), $KNbO_3$ (potassium niobate), BBO (beta-barium borate), LBO (lithium triborate), GaSe (gallium selenide), $ZnGeP_2$, and $LilO_3$ (lithium iodate).

Example: Nd-YAG laser normally emits a 1064 nm wavelength in harmonic generation, and can emit at

- 532 nm at second harmonic (green) – frequency doubling;

- 355 nm at third harmonics (UV) – frequency tripling; and

- 266 nm at fourth harmonics (ultraviolet) – frequency quadrupling.

1.2.3 Power

Laser generates high energy light. When focused, energy per unit area reaches extremely high levels, capable of damaging tissues, making them medically useful but potentially dangerous to work with.

Terminology	Description	Measurement unit	Symbol
Radiance	Laser energy measurement	Joules	J
Fluence	Laser energy per square meter	Joules/square metre	J/m^2
Power	All laser energy (transmitted, emitted, reflected) per unit time	Watt = joules/second	W
Irradiance or intensity	Laser power per square surface area	Watts/square metre	W/m^2
Power is measured in watts = Joules/sec (energy/time)			
Threshold power is the least power needed to obtain a just visible tissue effect. **Subthreshold energy** uses lower power, to achieve effects without visible burns.			
Power is modulated by altering energy or time **(P= E/t)**, so increasing laser energy or reducing pulse duration will increase laser power.			
Irradiance/power density = power/area = watts/cm^2. Increasing power or reducing spot size will increase power density, for a more intense effect.			

1.2.4 Mode

CW mode – Lasers emit continuous radiation and are more damaging than pulsed lasers due to longer tissue exposure. Emission >0.25 second is regarded as CW.

Pulsed mode – emissions occur in short bursts of highly concentrated energy.

- Pulses can be **long (millisecond), short (microsecond)**, Q-switched (**nanosecond –** extremely short pulse), or mode locked, emitting **picosecond pulses.**

- Number of pulses delivered per second is the **repetition rate**, which can vary from low (<1 pulse/second) to exceedingly high rates (>100/second)

- Solid-state lasers usually operate in the pulsed mode, to achieve higher power for photo-disruption with reduced risk of heat generation and collateral damage.

A CW laser can be made to operate in the pulsed mode, by

- modulating the pump to stimulate intermittently or

- modulating the output, to release intermittently, using locks and switches.

Modes of Laser Emission		
Laser mode	**Laser type**	**Wavelength**
CW – emits constant laser output from a constant pump source. Generates lower power than pulsed mode.	CO$_2$ laser **Argon**	10,600 nm 488 nm, 514 nm
Quasi CW – mechanical shutter produces bursts of CW output, or shorter pulses of milliseconds, with slightly higher energy.	KTP laser, **PASCAL** Copper bromide vapour laser Argon pumped tuneable dye laser Krypton laser	532 nm 510 nm, 514 nm 577 nm, 585 nm 568 nm
Pulsed mode – generate higher energy than CW output. **High energy – v. short pulse** The repetition rate can vary from short to long intervals.	Pulsed dye laser (PDL) Q-switched ruby laser Q-switched alexandrite laser **Q-switched Nd-YAG laser** PASCAL Er-YAG CO$_2$ pulsed laser	585–595 nm 694 nm 755 nm 1064 nm 532 nm 2940 nm 10,600 nm
Very short pulse laser (picosecond)	Nd-YAG Alexandrite laser	1064, 532 nm 755 nm

Generation of Pulsed Laser

- **Pulsed pumping** – Intermittent stimulation, using external switch/modulator (shutter).

- **Pulsed release** – internal modulation or switches that release laser intermittently.

Various techniques are used to alter pulse durations, allowing stored energy to be released as a giant pulse of extremely high energy, in a short pulse duration. Energy generated in a pulsed mode is much higher than a CW mode.

Device/technique to alter pulse duration	Laser pulse duration
Electronic shutters	1 ms
Pulsed flash lamps	1 us
Q-switching	1 ns
Mode locking	1 fs

Generation of pulsed laser – Turning the laser on and off by internal modulation is more efficient in generating higher energy, which is stored and released as a giant pulse when needed.

Gain switch	Q- Switch	Cavity dumping	Mode locking
Pulsed pumping (with flash lamp or another laser), using shutters or switches. Inefficient method. Generates lower power and longer pulses.	Q-switch blocks one mirror, preventing laser amplification, but pump continues to stimulate (energy stored as population inversion). When activated it generates high energy in a short pulse.	Both mirrors 100% reflective, allowing build-up and storage of high energy. Use crystals to diffract laser release via a different outlet (acoustic-optic deflectors, electro-optic modulators).	Uses constructive interference to mode lock or couple ultra-short pulses by altering resonant cavity length. It generates ultrashort pulses (picosecond and femtosecond) with a high repetition rate.

Generates less power – examples are Nd-YAG laser, Ti-Sapphire laser (can use cavity dumping, or q-switch or mode locking to generate pulse

Excimer laser Metal vapour laser	Nd-YAG laser	Generate less power than Q-switch.	Ti-Sapphire laser

Three Ways to Achieve Q-Switching

- Use mirror or prism rotating opposite to, but not aligned to the output mirror in the resonant cavity, preventing amplification. Periodically, alignment is achieved, producing a Q-switched pulse.

- Insertion of electro-optic or acoustic-optical device in the in the resonator cavity, which modulates the laser pathway and its release in short bursts.

- Insertion of a non-linear absorbent element in the cavity, which blocks one of the mirrors and only becomes transparent when a certain amount of energy is attained in the resonant cavity, generating a Q-switched pulse.

1.3 LASER DELIVERY SYSTEMS

Laser treatment can be delivered by various routes.

1. A **slit lamp Slit lamp – Contact lens contact lens is the commonest, safest, and most controlled method of laser delivery**, with a standardized spot size, due to a stable working distance.

2. **Indirect ophthalmoscopy with a +20D condensing lens.** Spot size varies, based on working distance and power of condensing lens.

3. **Trans scleral** – cyclodiode.

4. **Endo-laser** – during vitrectomy.

5. **Fundal camera-based delivery** (Navilas).

1.3.1 Slit Lamp Laser Delivery

The slit lamp is a high-powered, compound microscope with a long focal length, flexible slit-shaped illumination, and variable magnification, to provide a binocular, stereoscopic, and dynamic view of the eye. Accessory lenses (contact or non-contact) are used for fundal view. Contact lenses offer better control, focus spots, and improved laser safety.

Basics of slit lamp – a slit lamp has three main parts: mechanical system, illumination tower, and biomicroscope.

The mechanical system – provides coupling (common axis of rotation) of the microscope and illumination systems, which coincides with their focal plane (parfocality), to ensure that light will always fall where the microscope is focused.

The illumination system/tower – Consists of a light source, condensing lens, filters, horizontal and vertical slit diaphragms, projection lens, and reflecting mirror or prisms. Illumination comes from above (Haag Streit), or below (Zeiss), to provide a bright light, which is projected onto the eye under examination.

The illumination tower can be swivelled 180° on the horizontal axis and 20° on the vertical axis (slit lamp tilt). It houses filters, including:

■ Neutral density and heat absorption filter (reduces brightness and discomfort for photosensitive patients).

■ Cobalt blue filter (for tonometry, and corneal examination).

■ Red-free (green) filters enhance blood vessels and haemorrhages.

Biomicroscope observation system – Provides an enlarged, stereoscopic image of the eye. The LED filament is imaged on to the objective lens, but the mechanical slit is imaged on to the patient's eye – Kohler's Principle (ensures a bright beam with no glare).

The observation system comprises:

■ **Objective lens** – Two plano-convex lenses (power +22D and **telescope system** (between eye piece and objective lens) to alter magnification (Grenough flip lever ×10, ×16, or Galilean magnification wheel ×6, ×10, ×16, ×25, and ×40).

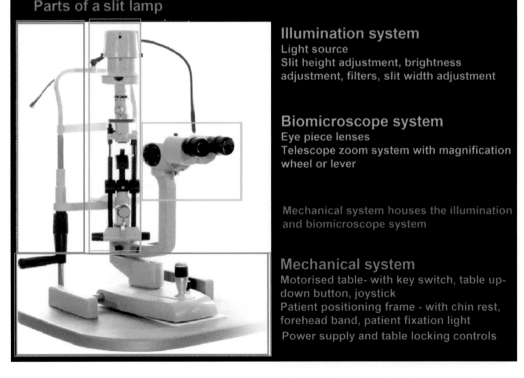

Figure 1.8 Parts of a slit lamp.

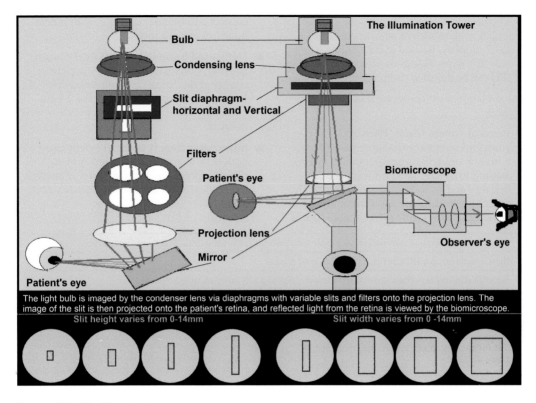

Figure 1.9 The illumination tower.

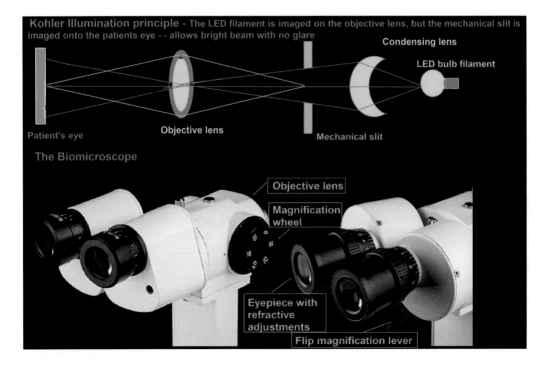

Figure 1.10 The biomicroscope.

- **Eyepiece lens** – Magnifying lenses (+10/+12D), with refractive adjustments from +7 to −7 dioptres, housed in converging tubes (10–16°), to provide good stereopsis. Eyepiece IPD can be adjusted, from 52mm to 78mm.

The slit lamp has three types of laser delivery systems:

- **Parfocal system (Zeiss, PASCAL)** – Slit lamp and laser have the same focal plane, with low beam divergence (parallel beam), leading to a sharp spot, uniform energy delivery and well-defined retinal burn. The size of the beam is the same at the cornea, lens, and retina, leading to potential risk of corneal or lenticular damage, with media opacities or poor focus.

- **Defocused beam delivery (Ellex)** – beam has high divergence, which reduces laser energy at the cornea and minimizes risk of inadvertent corneal burns. As the 2 focal planes are not the same, the spot is less well defined.

- **Surespot system (Lumenis)** – defocused system with a more controlled spot, to improve precision, reduce power density at the cornea, and increase laser efficacy and safety.

Slit lamp examination and laser treatment is preferably done in a semi-dark room
Adjust eyepieces, for IPD, refractive errors, and focus.

• Set **IPD slightly less than normal** to account for proximal convergence of slit lamp. • Set **a fraction more minus** than user refractive error to overcome proximal accommodation and convergence of the eyepieces. • **Set focus of eyepiece when first using slit lamp or laser.**	**Setting slit lamp eyepiece focus.** • *Use focusing rod (in slit lamp drawer). Mount it in front of microscope, by removing the flat groove alloy plate. Set slit beam 1–2mm wide and direct it at the centre of the rod.* • *Set one eyepiece at a time, by moving from the + side of scale, until the image first appears sharply focused (to avoid stimulating accommodation)* • *Make a note of the readings on the eyepiece and use this in the future. You do not need to use the focusing rod after this first occasion.*

• **Adjust table height** and chin rest for comfort. • Ensure slit beam is evenly illuminated with sharply demarcated edges. • **Pull joystick back and move slit lamp in to focus on area of interest. The final focus is sharpened by small movements of the joystick.**

Set Slit Parameters • **Slit brightness – Just visible level**. Excessive brightness causes glare, adversely affecting procedure and safety. • **Slit height – Tallest position** (remains unchanged during treatment). • **Slit width – moderate wide (5–6mm), keeping disc and fovea in view**. • **Narrow slit** – reduces FOV (smaller area of illumination) but increases depth of focus, useful to identify subtle details, treat mA, and sharpen focus. • **Wide slit** – allows larger FOV, good for faster treatment in PRP. • **Do not make the slit so narrow that you lose your bearings on the retina.**

Set slit lamp magnification **Low ×6 for initial examination and PRP** **High magnification ×10 or ×16 for details and FLT**

1.3.2 Binocular Indirect Ophthalmoscopy (BIO); Laser Indirect Ophthalmoscopy (LIO)

BIO offers good illumination, stereopsis, and FOV but lower magnification and can be difficult to learn. Movements affect size and clarity of the fundal image.

- **Fundal image is inverted and laterally transversed.**

- **Power of condensing lens determines retinal magnification and field of view.**

- **The 20D lens with working distance of 47mm provides a reasonable FOV, stereopsis, and magnification, and is the most common lens used.**

- **Fundal view and spot size are influenced by lens used, working distance, and patient's refractive error.**

Indirect ophthalmoscope-delivered laser (LIO) – For retinal vasculopathies and peripheral retinal diseases, in patients where slit lamp delivery is difficult (anxious, physically or mentally handicapped patients, paediatric patients, presence of media opacities, perioperative laser treatment after surgery). Patients lie supine – a lid speculum is used to keep the eye open and saline drops to keep the cornea moist.

LIO is a less controlled method of laser delivery, with no standardization of spot size and inability to treat the posterior pole safely.

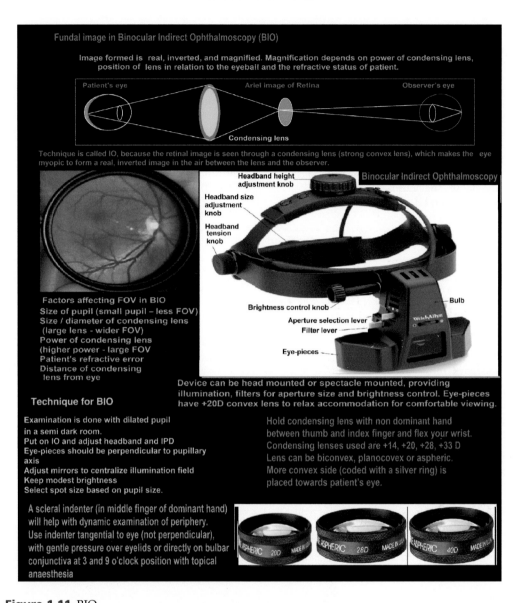

Figure 1.11 BIO.

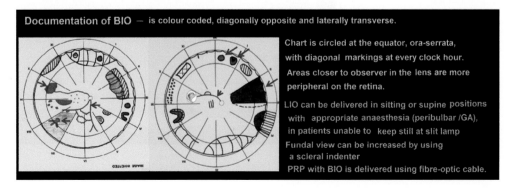

Figure 1.12 Documentation of BIO.

1.4 LASER TISSUE INTERACTION

Chromophores are pigments that absorb laser light to achieve tissue effect. The main ocular chromophores are melanin and haemoglobin. Understanding laser absorption spectrum of ocular tissues helps appropriate laser selection. (*Example: Blue lasers are not used for macular treatment. Red lasers can be used with macular haemorrhages.*)

Light falling on the retina is absorbed by melanin (RPE and choroid) and blood haemoglobin. The neurosensory retina is transparent and does not absorb laser wavelengths significantly. Laser effects (heating and coagulation) occur primarily in the pigmented outer retina.

The depth of penetration increases with longer wavelengths (red and IR) and absorption occurs more at the level of the choroid. Red krypton (647 nm) and the IR diode laser (810 nm) are absorbed mostly by choroidal melanocytes (only 8% RPE uptake).

Yellow krypton (568 nm) or diode (577 nm) are absorbed by oxyhaemoglobin, but not by xanthophyll pigment, making them useful in the treatment of juxta foveal microaneurysms and telangiectasias.

Chromophore (endogenous pigment)	Wavelengths absorbed optimally	Lasers used in practice
Melanin in RPE and Choroid	IR and visible spectrum (300–1300 nm)	Argon, PASCAL, Krypton laser
Haemoglobin (oxy and deoxyhaemoglobin)	Blue, green, and yellow (420–520 nm) (*red light is not absorbed*)	Argon, PASCAL, Krypton laser

Melanin absorbs green, yellow, and red wavelengths efficiently. Peak absorption is at 577 nm – yellow wavelength.
Oxy-haemoglobin in vascular tissues strongly absorbs 418, 542, and 577 nm (blue, green, yellow) wavelengths. Peak at 577 nm.

Xanthophyll – ocular pigment concentrated at the macula has maximum absorption of blue light and minimal absorption of red light. **A blue laser (Argon – 488 nm) should not be used in FLT, due to a high risk of macular burns (patients and doctor). Green, yellow, and red lasers are safer for treatment close to the macula.**

Water – IR lasers vaporize cellular and extracellular water to achieve effect (Nd-YAG, Diode, CO_2 lasers).

Exogenous pigments injected intravenously to accumulate in ocular tissues can also contribute in laser action, for example PDT.

Penetration of lasers – depends on wavelength and scattering. As wavelength increases, depth of penetration increases and scattering decreases. Visible ranges and near IR wavelengths penetrate tissues more than UV wavelengths.

Media opacity will increase scattering and reduce the laser effect.

Factors that affect laser – tissue interaction	
Laser variables: **Laser wavelength** (affects energy) **Spot size** (affects irradiance= power/area) **Laser power** (watts=energy/time) **Pulse duration** – affects power **Tissue variables:** **Tissue transparency** **Tissue pigmentation** **Tissue water content**	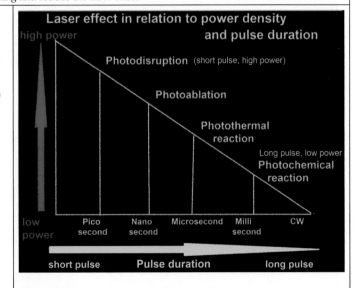

Figure 1.13 Laser effects in relation to power and pulse.

1.4.1 Principles of Laser Tissue Interactions

As irradiance (power) increases and pulse decreases, the effect varies from photochemical (at low power and long pulse) to photodisruption (high power and extremely short pulses).

Tissue effect	Irradiance=watts/cm²		Pulse duration=sec	
Photochemical effect	Low power		T >1 sec (CW)	
Photothermal	Slightly higher power		T <1 sec–1 μs	
Photoablation	Higher power		T <1 μs–1 ns	
Plasma induced ablation and photodisruption	Very high powers in a very small area		T <1 ns	

Photodisruption or Photoionization

Mechanical effect, with high-energy, short-pulse lasers. Causes optical breakdown of tissue molecules, generating a plume of plasma, which generates an acoustic shockwave that moves forwards to disrupt the target tissue nearby without any heat generation.
(Plasma is a pool of highly energized electrons that cause a precise optical breakdown.
Useful in breaking down tissues (YAG PI or capsulotomy), gallstones, or renal stones.)

Photoablation
• UV wavelengths (high-power lasers) break chemical or ionic bonds that hold tissues together, without heating, to cause clean-cut incisions. Excimer lasers in photorefractive keratectomy and Lasik.

Photovaporization
• When temperature rises to 60–100°C, cellular and extracellular water vaporize causing damage and disintegration, incision, and heat-related cauterization. Forms the basis of treatment in CO_2 and Femtolasers.

Photothermal
• Laser energy generates heat in target tissue, causing denaturation and coagulation of tissue proteins. The effect varies from **photocoagulation and photoevaporation to photocarbonization (charring)**, based on energy levels used
• Photothermal effect is utilized to cauterize blood vessels and weld tissues without sutures.
• Temperature rises of 10–20°C cause coagulation, protein denaturation, thrombus formation, and collagen contraction, and form the principle of PRP and FLT. Examples: argon, krypton, diode (810), and PASCAL lasers.

Photochemical
• Laser light triggers photochemical reaction (biostimulation) in target tissues to achieve therapeutic effects. Example: PDT, in treatment of ocular tumours and CNV.
• An exogenous photosensitizer (hematoporphyrin, benzoporphyrin) injected intravenously is selectively absorbed by blood vessels in metabolically active tissues such as CNV or tumours. When activated by a diode laser, the temperature rises and cytotoxic free oxygen radicals are released, to cause CNV destruction.

Photoradiation
• Laser light-generated cytotoxic effects to damage or kill cells. Dye lasers and wavelengths are absorbed by the injected dye to generate cytotoxic radicals.

1.4.2 Laser Mechanisms in the Retina

Ischaemia-driven vascular diseases, characterized by capillary non-perfusion and reduced oxygen availability, predominantly involve the inner retina. How does destroying the outer retina influence the inner retina?

The retina has a dual blood supply (retinal capillaries and choriocapillaris). Oxygen from choriocapillaris diffuses into the outer retina and is consumed by photoreceptors but does not reach the inner retina under normal circumstances.

Retinal vascular homeostasis is a balance between factors that promote neovascularization and leakage, and those that inhibit it. Hypoxia stimulates production of pro-inflammatory factors, cytokines, and angiogenic factors, such as VEGF, angiotensin II, leucocyte adhesion factor, inducing vasodilatation, and neovascularization. Retinal photocoagulation improves tissue oxygenation and reverses the consequences of hypoxia.

Retinal changes following laser photocoagulation
Laser energy absorbed by RPE heats retinal tissue causing scarring and pigment migration. Damage in the centre of the spot is greater than surrounding tissues (gaussian beam).

Temperature up to 42°C induces reversible changes – vasodilatation, release of chemical mediators, damage to intracellular organelle, endothelium, and reduced enzyme activity. New non-damaging, subthreshold lasers work in this region.

Temperature >50°C causes irreversible damage – cellular death reduces hypoxia and VEGF production, and increases production of PEDF. Current lasers work in this zone.

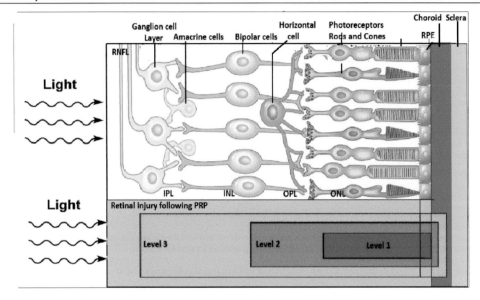

Figure 1.14 Retinal injury following PRP.

High energy, long exposure time and a large spot cause larger areas of retinal injury.
Level 1 – damage confined to choriocapillaris, RPE, and outer photoreceptors.
Level 2 – damage from choriocapillaris to outer nuclear and plexiform layers.
Level 3 – extends from deep choroid to ONL, IPL, and ganglion cell layer.

1.4.3 Starling's Law and Macular Oedema

Starling's law explains water exchange between vascular and extracellular tissue compartments in formation of vasogenic oedema, stating that

- If hydrostatic pressure = oncotic pressure – there is no movement between 2 compartments.

- If oncotic pressure > hydrostatic pressure, fluid will leak out, causing oedema.

- If hydrostatic pressure > oncotic pressure, it will drive fluid out, causing oedema.

Retinal arterioles are resistance vessels that control hydrostatic pressure downstream. **Diameter of retinal arterioles is controlled by oxygen levels**. In hypoxia, arterioles dilate, reducing resistance and increasing blood flow downstream, increasing the hydrostatic pressure, causing capillary dilatation and leakage. As fluid and proteins leak out, tissue oncotic pressure increases, attracting more fluid out and increasing the oedema. The process is controlled by VEGF, which in turn is influenced by oxygen levels.

1.4.4 How Does Focal Laser Treatment Reduce Macular Oedema?

The exact mechanism is unclear and likely to be multifactorial. It is established that **retinal blood flow and vessel diameters are inversely related to oxygen tension**. FLT increases retinal oxygenation, causing vasoconstriction, reducing blood flow, hydrostatic pressure, and oedema.

- **Direct coagulation of leaky capillaries** reduces vascular permeability and oncotic pressure.

- **Reduced hydrostatic pressure (improved oxygenation causing vasoconstriction).**

- **Improved RPE pump mechanism** to drain fluid. Regeneration and migration of surrounding healthy RPE cells, explains how gentle, subthreshold laser is effective.

- **Laser scars decrease local production of VEGF and inflammatory factors.**

Photothermal effects are dependent on:
Duration of laser action (pulse duration)   • **Longer exposure causes deeper tissue penetration and heat dissipation, leading to larger burns.** A CW laser causes more scarring than pulsed laser. Reducing pulse duration shortens treatment time, reduces pain, and minimizes scarring.   • **Thermal relaxation time (TRT)** is time taken for tissue to dissipate 60% of absorbed energy. Pulse duration <TRT vaporizes intracellular water (no time for heat diffusion), causing an explosive effect, with rupture of Bruch's membrane, and occurs with use of very high energy with an extremely short pulse.
Power density or irradiance (mW/cm^2)   Increasing laser power or reducing spot size results in increased power density, with increased thermal effects.
Photoreceptors are mitochondria-rich, high oxygen-consuming cells. Destroying them is an effective way of reducing oxygen consumption in the outer retina, allowing choroidal oxygen flux to reach the inner retina, improving hypoxia, and reducing neovascularization.   **A typical PRP session reduces photoreceptors and oxygen consumption of outer retina by approximately 20%.**
Improved oxygenation   • **Reduced demand** – photoreceptors have high metabolic activity and oxygen demand. PRP destroys them, reducing oxygen requirement.   • **Improved availability** – loss of some photoreceptors, improves oxygen supply to remaining photoreceptors, reducing hypoxic drive for angiogenesis.   • **Oxygen bridges** – loss of photoreceptors at site of laser allows oxygen flux from the choroid to travel through glial scars to the inner retina.   • **Vasoconstriction, reduced leakage** – improved oxygenation and direct coagulation of mA.
Reversal of angiogenic drive   • PRP reduces angiogenic burden by removing ischaemic retina from the equation. This reduces release of angiogenic factors (VEGF reduced by 70% after PRP).   • Remaining healthy retina produces anti-angiogenic factors.

Angiogenic factors that promote NV	Anti-angiogenic factors that inhibit NV
VEGF – vascular endothelial growth factor SDF-1 – stromal cell derived factor. PDGF – platelet derived growth factor Ang-2 – angiopoietin 2 EPO – erythropoietin Cytokines and multiple growth factors (TNF, Integrin)	PEDF – pigment epithelium derived factor TIMP3 – tissue inhibitor metalloproteinase 3 Endostatins Angiotensin TSP – Thrombospondin

Long-term effects of laser treatment
Gene regulations provide sustained effects. (Increased expression of genes related to healing and repair of organelles, inhibition of angiogenesis and axonal growth promotion, and reduced gene expression of angiogenic and inflammatory factors).

Gene upregulation	Gene downregulation	Repair / regeneration	RPE stimulation
Improve photoreceptor metabolism, cell renewal/remodelling. Increase axonal growth and synaptic function. Increased heat shock protein (HSP), increase matrix metalloproteinases (MMP) for structural repair. Increase TSP-1, Agtr2 anti-angiogenic factors.	Decrease endothelial proliferation/ dysfunction. Decrease angiogenic and vascular permeability factors (Fibroblast Growth factor-FG14, FG16), IL-1, plasminogen activator inhibitor-2, inhibitors of MMPs, calcitonin like receptor (CLR).	Activation, migration polarization, and phagocytic activity of microglia. Injured photoreceptor releases endothelin and activates Muller cells, leukocyte infiltration. RPE healing, and migration over treated area.	Gentle laser with short pulses and sub-threshold treatment causes thermal stress (photo-stimulation). Promotes cell repair and remodelling. Anti-angiogenic, anti-inflammatory, Neuroprotective effects.

1.5 LASER HAZARD AND LASER SAFETY PROTOCOLS

Lasers are associated with potential hazards for patients and clinicians, and laser safety is paramount to avoid laser related accidents.

The hazards relate to phototoxicity from high radiance (brightness) and high irradiance (ability to be focused into a small spot of concentrated energy), making lasers extremely dangerous to work with.

Visible and near IR light (400–1400 nm wavelength) can penetrate ocular media, causing retinal damage. UV and IR wavelengths (<400 nm and >1400 nm) are absorbed by the cornea and lens, causing corneal burns and cataracts. IR wavelengths are particularly dangerous, as they do not stimulate the protective blink reflex. Skin injury is more likely with prolonged exposure. UV rays cause sunburn type injury, while visible and IR rays cause thermal damage.

The extent of injury depends on laser wavelength, energy, exposure time, spot size, and target tissue factors (reflectivity, absorption, dispersion, and thermal properties). Short wavelengths and short pulses equate to higher energy with higher risk of injuries.

1.5.1 Laser Classification and Safety (ANSI Standards)

Lasers' safety is classified by their wavelengths and their maximum output power.

Classification of lasers – based on accessible emission limits (AEL) – *maximum power (watts) or energy (joules) that can be emitted in a specified wavelength range and exposure time.*	
Class 1 lasers	Safe under all conditions, due to low output or enclosed laser – no risk of exposure. Example: CD player, laser printer
Class 2 lasers	Associated with exposure to very bright light. Output power is up to 1 mw. Relatively safe because blink reflex reduces exposure to <0.25 sec. If blink reflex was supressed or patient stared into laser light, eye injury can occur. Example: supermarket scanner, laser light toys.
Class 3 lasers	**3A lasers** – output power is up to 2.5 mw, dangerous if used with optical instruments that focus light and increase power density. Examples: Laser pointers, laser sight on firearms. **3B lasers** – output is 5–500 mw. Dangerous if enters the eye, protective eyewear recommended, risk of skin burns, fire hazard. Diffuse reflection is safe, but specular reflection is dangerous.
Class 4 lasers	Power output >500 mw, high risk of ocular and skin injury, dangerous with both specular and diffuse reflections. Includes all industrial, scientific, military, and medical lasers. Protective eyewear recommended.
MPE – maximum permissible exposure – highest irradiance (power density w/cm^2), or fluence (energy density – J/cm^2) of light that is considered safe, measured at the cornea at a given wavelength and exposure time. It is usually 10% of the dose causing damage 50% of the time. MPE for UV and IR rays > visible rays, with a higher risk of injury.	

Laser hazards are classified as non-beam and beam related hazards.

Ocular injury can be reversible or permanent. Inadvertent exposure causes headache, lacrimation, gritty sensation, floaters, sudden visual loss with macular burn, or gradual loss from cataract, reduced retinal sensitivity, and colour vision.

Skin injuries – photochemical effects of mid/far UV rays cause sunburns, reddening, blisters, premature ageing, and skin cancers (UV – 290–320 nm). Thermal burns are rare – they occur with high energy and prolonged exposure (CO_2 and some IR lasers). **There is a higher risk of burns in photosensitive patients (idiopathic or drug related).**

Non beam related hazards – safety related to:	
Laser path	Avoid reflectors – jewellery, metal fittings, mirrors. Avoid absorbers – trapped eyelash, mascara. Avoid flammables – oxygen cylinder, cleaning solution, chemicals.
Unregulated equipment	Unregulated laser pointers, toys available on the internet, may cause ocular injury with flash blindness. Regulations may vary in countries.
Electrical hazards	Lasers are high voltage devices with electrical and fire hazards. Risk is higher during maintenance and servicing. Ensure cables are not frayed and floor is not wet.
Chemical hazards	Chemicals in lasing media can be toxic/hazardous substances, dyes, flammable solvents, heavy metal vapours. Toxic plume (dust, metallic, chemical, biologic fumes) can contaminate the air with industrial lasers. Room must be well ventilated, and protective masks may be used.
Mechanical hazards	Explosions, laser leakage from damaged cables, unstable table. Periodic checks and laser maintenance are essential.

Beam-related hazards	
Wavelength ranges	Pathological effects
180–315 nm (UV-B, UV-C)	Photokeratitis, corneal inflammation, erythema, increased skin pigmentation, accelerated skin aging, skin cancer
315–400 nm (UV-A)	Photochemical cataract, skin pigmentation, skin burns
400–780 nm (visible light)	Photothermal retinal injury, skin pigmentation, light photosensitivity, cataract, skin burn
780–1400 nm (near IR)	Cataract, retinal burn, skin burn
1400–3000 nm (IR) >3000 nm (far IR)	Aqueous flare, cataract, corneal burn, skin burn
Type of beam exposure **Direct exposure or indirect exposure** (reflections from grade 4 lasers). **Specular reflection** – from flat reflectors (mirror) – risk of harm is high. **Diffuse reflection** – from irregular reflectors (jewellery, metal tools) – lower risk of harm. A surface may be a diffuse reflector for one, but specular for another wavelength.	
Factors that affect laser hazards	
Laser parameters	
Wavelength (determines energy and absorption)	UV rays (180–390 nm), mid-far IR (1400 nm–1 mm) – corneal and lens injury. Visible and near IR (400–1400 nm) penetrates ocular media, absorbed by the retina and macula. **Maximum retinal absorption is at 400–570 nm, making Argon and PASCAL lasers hazardous for eye injuries.**
Energy	Higher energy – higher risk of injury. Shorter wavelength (UV) has higher energy than longer (IR) wavelengths.
Spot size	Smaller spot (focused laser) has higher energy density with higher risk of injury, especially if used with high energy. (Reduce power with small spots.)
Pulse duration	A short pulse is associated with a risk of photomechanical injury, while a long pulse is associated with photothermal injury (longer exposure).
Pulse Repetition	Faster rate – associated with less heat dissipation and phototoxicity.
Eye factors – the biconvex lens acts as a magnifier and focuses laser light on the retina. Even a low-powered laser or diffuse laser reflection can cause retinal injury.	
Self-defence mechanisms – blink reflex, light aversion, and head turn protect against visible light. UV and IR lasers do not stimulate the blink reflex and can be harmful. Sustained exposure with laser pointer directed at an eye can cause injury. **Size of pupil** – small pupil is associated with lesser exposure. **Degree of pigmentation** in target tissue – dark fundi have a higher risk of injury. **Aphakia and Pseudophakia** – aphakes have a clear media and pseudophakic IOL focuses laser light, increasing the risk of injury.	

1.5.2 Laser Safety Protocols
Know Your Laser Safety Officer in the Hospital.
Ensure treatment is performed in a controlled environment, to mitigate laser hazards.

Laser Room

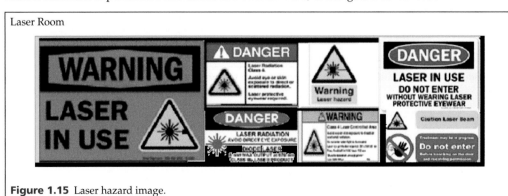

Figure 1.15 Laser hazard image.

Best practice in the laser eye clinic
Always laser in a controlled area – dedicated room, proper ventilation, and sign-posted.
Switch on the red warning light outside the door, to ensure the **room becomes a restricted area** and prevent inadvertent entry.
Do not open the door while the laser is operational. The room may be locked during use, although this may hinder access in case of an emergency. **Knock and wait for the operator to allow entry** (the laser can be stopped temporarily, if entry is essential).
When the treatment session is finished, switch off the laser and red light, remove/return key to the nurse.
Laser machine, users, and maintenance – Familiarize yourself with machine, procedure, and hazards. Treatment should only be done by trained and authorized users.
Always switch on and off with the key, not the emergency button.
Always keep the laser in stand-by mode, until ready for treatment – This prevents inadvertent laser emission as the safety shutter is closed (activated in ready mode).
Do not leave the room unattended with the key in situ. Keep the laser on standby, shut the door, or ask a nurse to keep watch, if leaving the room for a short period.
Keep people in the room to the minimum (2–4) – doctor, patient, nurse if help required, relative (anxious, young patients, language barrier, disability). All in the laser room must wear appropriate, undamaged safety glasses (except doctor – protected by inbuilt filters).
Use a wheel lock to prevent excessive movement; do not trap wires, put anything heavy on the table, or raise the table too high – risk of toppling.
Laser maintenance – ensure the laser is protected when not in use. • The machine should be serviced once a year, including slit lamp focus, aiming beam focus, laser parameters and bodywork – table movement and stability. • Do not use the laser if you see error codes/messages on the display screen– switch off and on again. If the error persists – inform the laser safety officer.
Laser treatment – Do not laser if view not clear, aiming beam not visible, error codes seen, or there is excessive patient movement. Document error codes for manufacturer reference.
Use just visible illumination and complete treatment in the shortest time (reduce phototoxicity).
Always perform laser with appropriate lenses – stabilizes eye and improves safety.
Use threshold power – least power needed to get just visible effect. **Use a smaller spot, shorter pulse duration, and smaller grids.**
If patient complains of pain – reduce the exposure time, laser power, grid size, or use a magnifying CL. Consider 2× paracetamols 1 hour prior to treatment or pre-laser sub-tenon/peribulbar anaesthesia, or LIO with GA in patients with low pain threshold.
Seek help with anxious patients or difficult cases. Preparation is key.
Document treatment parameters, including adverse events or potential difficulties for future reference and treatment planning.
Dealing with emergency hazards: **Patient related emergency** – fainting, fits, collapse. **Use the emergency stop button (stops laser immediately), call for help, then see to the patient.** Do not use the emergency stop button unless necessary. Key ignition will not work if the button is activated. Press it again to deactivate it.
Fire alarm – do not panic. Stop treatment. The nurse should take the patient to a safe area. **Switch off normally** at the machine and mains. Remove key, and evacuate room. A fire extinguisher should be handy/available.
Water leak – do not use the laser until it is checked and declared safe for use by engineers.
An incident report should always be filled with details of the adverse event. Guidance is provided by the laser safety officer and the health board 'Health and Safety officer'.

1.5.3 Laser Safety Eyewear

Lasers are extremely bright sources of EMR (electromagnetic radiation), with a risk of permanent ocular injury without suitable protection, particularly during inspection of delivery system.

Risk of Eye Damage • **Visible and near infrared wavelengths – retinal damage** • **UV and IR wavelengths – corneal and scleral damage** • **Prescription glasses – concentrates laser energy, worsening the damage.**

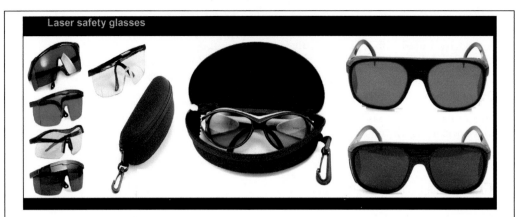

Figure 1.16 Laser safety glasses.

Reducing beam related hazards with protective eyewear:
- Glasses with appropriate filters protect eyes from direct or reflected laser light.
- A **coloured filter** should be selected to prevent transmission of the relevant wavelength. (*Example: Orange filter absorbs 532nm, but transmits wavelengths >550nm, useful with argon laser, but not with a diode laser, 800nm.*)
- Eyewear is also rated for **optical density**, which quantifies the amount of light transmitted. They reduce beam power below MPE and reduce risk of ocular exposure, but also reduce vision in general.
- Eyewear should also be able to withstand direct laser exposure without breaking.

The ANSI Z136.1 standard	
Eyewear not recommended	**Eyewear recommended**
Class 1 laser – not hazardous Class 1M lasers (visible 400–700 nm), used without magnifying optics Class 2 lasers – visible lasers safe with blink reflex of 0.25 sec	Class 2M – visible (400–700nm) Class 3R – MPE ×5 for class 2 visible laser, or ×5 for class 1 invisible lasers (high risk) Class 3 B – high risk from direct exposure Class 4 – from direct and diffuse exposure

Safety glasses must be used by all in the room, except doctor (protected by filters).
Glasses must be wavelength specific and appropriately labelled.

Glasses colour	Suitable wavelength	Used with lasers
Orange	450–532 nm (visible)	Argon, KTP lasers
Magenta	500–600 nm (visible)	Freq-doubled YAG, PASCAL
Pink	720–830 nm (near IR)	Alexandrite, diode lasers
Green	1064 nm (IR)	YAG laser
Clear Glass	10600 nm (far IR) 190–360 nm (UV)	CO_2 laser Excimer laser

Optical density filter – dictates how much light is transmitted through the glasses. Varies from 0 (100% transmission) to 7 (0.00001% transmission) of laser light. OD of 3 allows 0.1% transmission and offers good protection, without affecting vision. Higher OD will blur the user's vision.

The laser machine has an inbuilt filter to protect the operator from exposure.

Safety eyewear needed is based on Maximum Permissible Exposure (MPE), Nominal Ocular Hazard Area (NOHA), and Nominal Ocular Hazard Distance (NOHD) for each delivery device and configuration of treatment room. For additional information, refer to the laser device's user manual and international laser standards and guidelines.

1.6 LASER LENSES

An emmetropic eye emits parallel rays from the fundus and cannot be examined at a short distance. Contact lenses allow examination by creating an intermediate fundal image within the focal plane of the slit lamp.

Lenses are essential tools for safe laser delivery. The contact lens and eye work together as a single optical system to improve visualization and facilitate therapeutic intervention.

1.6.1 Advantages of Contact Lenses in Lasers

Laser treatment without the magnifying and focusing mechanisms of lenses is less controlled, requiring higher power, with increased risk of damage to surrounding tissues.

Contact lenses, used with topical anaesthesia and coupling lubricant:

■ Act as a speculum, keeping eyes moist and lids out of the way.

■ Stabilize the eye (prevents blink reflex and reduce ocular movements).

■ Focus laser spots precisely on target areas.

■ Some lenses magnify (useful in FLT), while others offer wide FOV (beneficial in PRP).

■ Reduce laser hazards and surrounding tissue damage.

1.6.2 Safety Principles of Contact Lenses

Laser power and energy density are inversely proportional to spot size.

The spot is responsible for target effect (cutting efficiency, thermal burns) and volume of tissue affected.

Small spots deliver more concentrated energy, and therefore require less power to achieve effects. Conversely, a large spot requires higher energy for similar tissue effect, with reduced laser safety.

1.6.3 Laser Cone Angle

Laser beams converge to and diverge beyond a point of focus, forming a cone angle (angle of convergence and divergence). The sharper the focus and smaller the spot (point of focus), the larger the cone angle. The spot size has an inverse relationship to the cone angle.

Unfocused spot without CL	Focused spot with CL
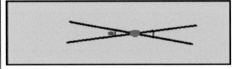	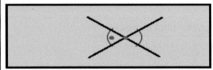
Unfocused spot is large with smaller cone angle. This means that the laser energy is still concentrated around the spot, with a higher risk of damage to surrounding tissues (purple dot).	*Focused spot is small and cone angle is large. Laser beam diverges quickly before and after the focused spot, reducing risk of damage to surrounding tissues*

- Cone angle is related to laser safety. A CL focuses the spot sharply, increasing the cone angle, with sharp divergence of laser beam before and after, reducing laser concentration around the spot.
- A large cone angle means a small, focused spot with more intense tissue effects. This:
  - **Reduces laser energy requirement.**
  - **Reduces risk of collateral damage, and increases laser safety.**

1.6.3.1 Optical Characteristics of Ocular Media

Alteration in optical characteristics of the media (e.g. after vitreous surgery) can affect RI of the eye/, create multiple interfaces, affecting, focus, magnification, and laser parameters (spot size, power density), resulting in suboptimal treatment.

The size of the spot is directly proportional to wavelength in vacuum (spot size increases with increasing wavelength) and inversely to RI of the medium (spot size reduces with increasing refractive indices of a medium).

The spot size reduces as the laser beam moves from air into the eye (RI > 1), aided further by using CL.

- **Phakic eye – air in cavity** (RI of 1.00) – Increases posterior lens convexity, increasing lens power significantly (myopic shift).

- **Aphakic eye with air** – posterior corneal surface changes from a weak concave to a strong concave lens, neutralizing the power of the anterior cornea, allowing a fundal view without any optical aides/lenses.

- **Phakic eye with silicone oil** – RI of silicone oil > normal lens, so silicone oil acts as a concave lens on the posterior lens surface (normally a weak convex lens), making it into a weak concave (negative) lens – **hypermetropic shift.**

- **Aphakic eye with silicone oil** – the posterior corneal surface is normally a low-power concave lens. Silicone oil in the cavity acts as a convex lens at the posterior corneal surface causing a slight myopic shift.

- **Pseudophakia with a flat posterior surface IOL** – no change, as flat surfaces do not have any refractive power.

1.6.4 Lens Classification

Lenses are classified into anterior and posterior segment lenses.

- **Anterior segment lenses** are used to visualize lens capsule, IOL, and ocular angle.

- **Posterior segment lenses** are used to visualize vitreous and retina. They are further classified as:

  - **Concave CL (negative lens)** – creates an **upright, virtual fundal image**

  - **Convex lens (positive lens)** – creates an **inverted, real fundal image**

  - **Mirror lens**

1.6.5 Common Features of Laser Contact Lenses

- Concave posterior surface (conforms to corneal curvature, for a comfortable fit).

- Flat, convex, or concave anterior surface, or planar mirrors, allow tissue visualization.

- PMMA shell with knurled edges to facilitate lens manipulation.

- Flanges to stabilize the eye and prevent blinking.

- Anti-reflective coating on lens surface reduces glare and laser hazards. *Hazard distance is reduced from 7 metres to 1.6 metres for coated lenses. Anti-reflective coating reduces reflected light from 4% to 1%.*

Contact lenses used in photothermal laser treatment			
	Concave lenses	Convex lenses	Mirror lenses
Image	Erect, upright, virtual	Inverted, real	Laterally transverse image
FOV	Less	Wide FOV	FOV increased by rotation
Magnification	High	Low	High
Examples	Goldmann (−67D), Hruby (−58.6D)	Mainster, Volk, panfundoscope	Goldmann 3-mirror lens

Convex lenses and the 3-mirror lens are used most often in clinical practice.

Lens name	Lens type (anterior surface)	Image	Lens power (approx.)	Magnifi-cation	FOV^0 static – dynamic	Spot magnification	Burn with 200 μm spot	Uses
Mainster M. Focal Mx1 M-165	Biconvex aspheric	Real inverted	+61 +90 +115	×0.96 ×0.68 ×0.51	90–121 118–127 165–180	×1.05 ×1.50 ×1.96	210 μm 300 μm 392 μm	FLT PRP PRP, pexy
Quad Superquad	Biconvex aspheric	Real inverted	+115 +120	×0.51 ×0.5	120–144 160–165	×1.97 ×2.0	394 μm 400 μm	PRP, pexy
Panfundoscope	Convex spheric	Real inverted	+85	×0.71	160–170	×1.41	282 μm	PRP
Area centralis	Biconvex aspheric	Real inverted	+60	×0.93	70-84	×0.94	188 μm	FLT
Volk widefield	Biconvex aspheric	Real inverted	+120	×1.08	160–170	×2.0	400 μm	PRP
Goldmann 3-mirror	Flat, mirror	Mirror image	Mirror	×0.93	360° rotation	×1.08	216 μm	PRP, pexy

Wide field lens – Mainster-165, Volk Quad, Superquad, HR wide field, panfundoscope

Advantages – wide FOV, greater working distance, lens rotation not required. Good for retinal orientation and quick PRP.
Disadvantages – minified view, difficult to see fundal details and laser burns clearly. **Spot size doubles, causing larger burns. Do not use spot >200 μm with widefield lenses.** A 200 μm spot delivers a 400 μm burn, and a 400 μm spot delivers an 800 μm burn, causing large scars. **In addition, as spot size doubles, laser energy required increases ×4, making treatment painful and increasing laser hazards.**

How to select laser lenses appropriately: Selection depends on treatment planned, user experience, and patient's refractive error.

Focal/grid laser	Mid-peripheral PRP or retinopexy	Complete PRP/far peripheral PRP or Retinopexy
• **Mainster focal** • **Area centralis**	• **Mainster ×1** • **Goldmann 3-mirror broad mirror**	• **Mainster-165** • **3-mirror tall mirror** • **Volk Quad/Superquad**

- Wide-angled lenses offer good view of entire fundus, allowing quick PRP, but double spot size, minify view by 50%, and increase energy requirement by ×4.
- **Patient's refractive errors, will influence fundal magnification, except with 3-mirror lens. Myopia – increased magnification, reduced FOV** (widefield or 3-mirror lens good).
- **Hypermetropia – decreased magnification, increased FOV** (3-mirror lens better).
- Concave lenses increase degree of myopia and shorten working distance – **patients with a high degree of pre-existing myopia – select a convex lens or a 3-mirror lens**.
- **Mainster ×1 is ideal for training, and mid-peripheral PRP** (*good FOV + higher magnification*).
- **Select Volk Quad or Superquad with small eyes (PA) and small pupils.**

1.6.6 Lens Used with YAG Laser

Stabilizes the eye, magnifies view, aids precise focus on PCO or iris, and reduces risk of IOL pits or corneal burn, by increasing cone angle.

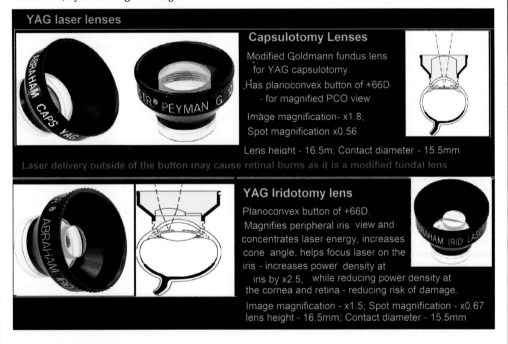

Figure 1.17 YAG laser lenses.

Gonioscopy – Light emanating from the angle undergoes total internal reflection (TIR) and is normally not visible. The critical angle for the cornea–air interface is 45°, and light from the angle needs to strike the cornea steeper than the critical angle to be visible.

RI of goniolens = RI of the cornea, eliminating cornea–air interface and allowing light to emerge at the new lens–air interface, at a steeper angle, allowing direct visualization.

Direct gonioscopy – not commonly used

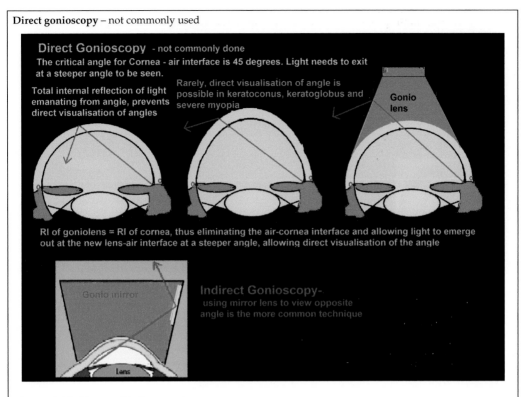

Figure 1.18 Direct and indirect gonioscopy.

Indirect gonioscopy with mirrors is a more common technique – view opposite angle.

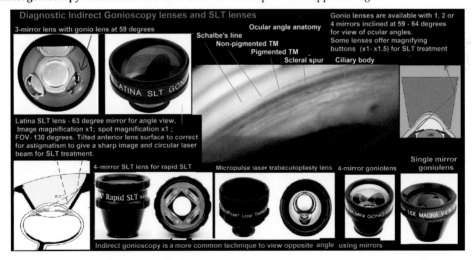

Figure 1.19 Gonioscopy and SLT lenses.

3-mirror lens – higher magnification, good for peripheral PRP and retinopexies – better view and laser burn visibility than wide field lenses.

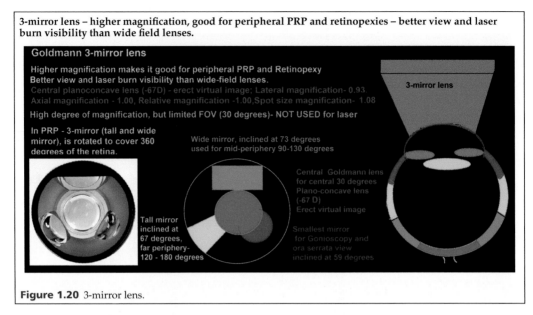

Figure 1.20 3-mirror lens.

1.6.7 Contact Lenses Used in Conjunction with Photothermal Lasers

CL offer benefits, with improved view, high magnification, wide FOV, and improved safety.

1.6.7.1 Common Contact Lenses Used in the Laser Clinic

1.6.7.1.1 Mainster Lenses for Laser

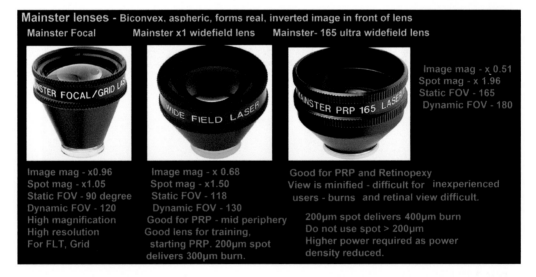

Figure 1.21 Mainster lenses.

1.6.7.2 Volk Lenses for Laser

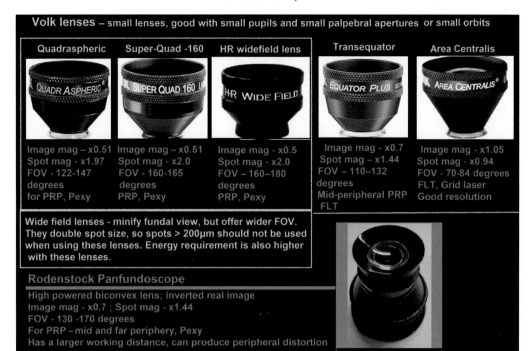

Volk lenses – small lenses, good with small pupils and small palpebral apertures or small orbits

Quadraspheric	Super-Quad -160	HR widefield lens	Transequator	Area Centralis
Image mag – x0.51 Spot mag - x1.97 FOV - 122-147 degrees for PRP, Pexy	Image mag – x0.51 Spot mag - x2.0 FOV - 160-165 degrees PRP, Pexy	Image mag - x0.5 Spot mag - x2.0 FOV – 160-180 degrees PRP, Pexy	Image mag - x0.7 Spot mag – x1.44 FOV – 110–132 degrees Mid-peripheral PRP FLT	Image mag - x1.05 Spot mag - x0.94 FOV - 70-84 degrees FLT, Grid laser Good resolution

Wide field lenses - minify fundal view, but offer wider FOV. They double spot size, so spots > 200µm should not be used when using these lenses. Energy requirement is also higher with these lenses.

Rodenstock Panfundoscope

High powered biconvex lens; inverted real image
Image mag - x0.7 ; Spot mag - x1.44
FOV - 130 -170 degrees
For PRP – mid and far periphery, Pexy
Has a larger working distance, can produce peripheral distortion

Figure 1.22 Volk lenses.

1.6.7.3 Indirect Ophthalmoscopy

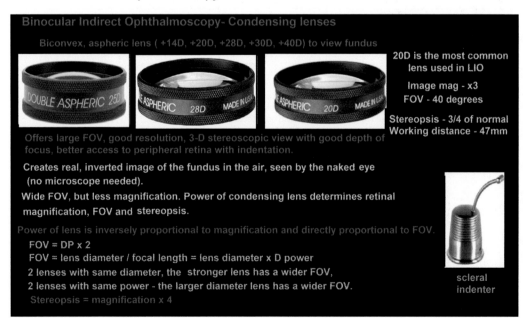

Binocular Indirect Ophthalmoscopy- Condensing lenses

Biconvex, aspheric lens (+14D, +20D, +28D, +30D, +40D) to view fundus

20D is the most common lens used in LIO

Image mag - x3
FOV - 40 degrees

Stereopsis - 3/4 of normal
Working distance - 47mm

Offers large FOV, good resolution, 3-D stereoscopic view with good depth of focus, better access to peripheral retina with indentation.

Creates real, inverted image of the fundus in the air, seen by the naked eye (no microscope needed).

Wide FOV, but less magnification. Power of condensing lens determines retinal magnification, FOV and stereopsis.

Power of lens is inversely proportional to magnification and directly proportional to FOV.

FOV = DP x 2
FOV = lens diameter / focal length = lens diameter x D power
2 lenses with same diameter, the stronger lens has a wider FOV,
2 lenses with same power - the larger diameter lens has a wider FOV.

Stereopsis = magnification x 4

scleral indenter

Figure 1.23 BIO lenses.

1.6.7.3.1 How Does Refractive Error Affect Fundal View?

Refractive power of an emmetropic eye is approximately +60D.
Patient's refractive error affects image magnification and laser spot size.

Magnification of image = <u>Refractive power of eye × slit lamp magnification</u>
                                Dioptre power of the contact lens used

Emmetropia – ref power of eye = 60D	×10 slit lamp mag	×16 slit lamp mag
+60D lens	10	16
+78D lens	7.7	12.3
+90D lens	6.6	10.6

Hyperopia of +10D - ref power of eye = 50D			Myopia of −10D – ref power of eye = 70D		
Slit lamp magnification	×10	×16	Slit lamp magnification	×10	×16
A +60D lens – magnifies	8.33	13.33	A + 60D lens – magnifies	11.65	18.66
A +78D lens – magnifies	6.4	10.26	A +78D lens – magnifies	8.97	14.36
A +90D lens – magnifies	5.55	8.89	A +90D lens – magnifies	7.78	12.44

Fundal view is magnified in myopia
Fundal view is minified in hypermetropia

Principles of image magnification also apply to laser lenses. The fundal view is magnified in myopes and minified in hypermetropes. Keep this in mind when selecting contact lenses for treatment.

Fundal magnification is not affected by refractive errors with a 3-mirror lens.

Lens parameters
- **Magnification of lens = dioptre/4**
- **Magnification of retina = dioptre power of eye/dioptre power of lens**
- **Retinal mag on slit lamp = <u>dioptre power of eye × slit lamp magnification</u>**
                                    dioptre power of lens
- **Stereopsis = magnification/4**
- **Field of view = dioptre power of lens × 2**
- Magnification is inversely proportional to lens power and working distance, and directly proportional to lens diameter.
- If lens power is the same, a larger lens will provide a wider FOV.
- If lens diameter is the same, the higher power lens has a larger FOV, but lower magnification.

Lens	Mag power	Retinal mag	Stereopsis	FOV	Usefulness
+30D	×7 (30/4)	×2 (60/30)	0.5 (7/4)	60°	Panoramic view Working dist – 26 mm, not good for PRP
+20D	×5 (20 /4)	×3	0.75	40°	Working dist – 47 mm, good for laser
+15D	×3.75	×4	1.0	30°	Good for disc/macula

- **Axial ametropia** – image smaller in hyperopia and **larger in myopia by 2%/dioptre of error.**
- **Refractive ametropia** – image smaller in hyperopia, larger in myopia by 0.5%/dioptre of error.
- **Myopes** – larger image (increased magnification, stereopsis, reduced FOV).
- **Hyperopes** – smaller image (reduced magnification, stereopsis, larger FOV).
- **BIO** – changing working distance can compensate for patient refractive error, so in practice refractive error does not affect the retinal image with IO.
  - **Moving closer will magnify the image but reduce FOV.**
  - **Moving away will minify the image but increase FOV.**

SUGGESTED READING

1. Thomas, G. et al. Basic principles of lasers. *Anaesthesia and Intensive Care Medicine* 2011;12(12):574–577, https://doi.org/10.1016/j.mpaic.2011.09.013

2. *Laser – principles of working laser, understanding the basics | lasers | photonics handbook,* www.physics-and-radio-electronics.com/physics/laser/principles…(rp-photonics.com)

3. Jacques, S.L. Laser-tissue interactions. Chemical, thermal, mechanical. *Surg Clin North Am.* 1992;72(3):531–558.

4. Jennings, P.E. et al. Oxidative effects of laser photocoagulation. *Free Radical Biol Med.* 1991;11:327–330.

5. *Guidance on safe use of lasers, ILSS and LEDs in medical, surgical, dental, and anaesthetic practices, DB2008(03) April 2008, Medicines and Healthcare products Regulatory Agency,* ISBN 9781-90- 073165-7

6. Mainster, M.A. et al. Retinal laser lenses: magnification, spot size, and FOV. *Br J Ophth.* 1990;74(3):177–179.

7. Laser lenses. From www.ocularinc.com/_data/product/

8. Mizuno, K. Binocular indirect argon laser photocoagulator. *Br J Ophthalm.* 1981;65(6):425–428.

9. Fankhauser, F. et al. Optical aids and their application. *Int Ophthalmol Clin.* 1990;30(2):123–129.

10. Jain, A. et al. Effect of pulse duration on retinal photocoagulation. *Arch Ophthalmol.* 2008;126(1):78–85.

11. Binz, N. et al. Long-term effect of laser photocoagulation on gene expression. *FASEB J.* 2006;20(2):383–385.

12. Ogata, N. et al. Upregulation of PEDF after laser photocoagulation. *Am J Ophthalmol.* 2001; Sep;132(3):427–429.

13. Romero-Aroca, P. et al. DME pathophysiology: vasogenic vs inflammatory. *J Diabetes Res.* 2016; Article ID 2156273, http://dx.doi.org/10.1155/2016/2156273.

14. Satirtav, G. et al. Current evidence of pathophysiology of DME: a review. *World J Ophthalmol.* 2014;4:147–151.

Section 2 YAG Laser

This section deals with the YAG laser machine and common YAG laser procedures in the eye clinic, with a basic understanding of underlying pathology, diagnosis, approach to management, and appropriate laser parameters for treatment.

2.1 THE ND-YAG LASER

The Nd-YAG is a class 3b solid state laser, using an Yttrium-Aluminium-Garnet crystal, doped with neodymium – the active lasing medium.

When optically pumped by a diode laser, it emits light in the near IR wavelength (1064 nm). It can also emit at 532 nm (visible light) using a KTP crystal, for SLT and photothermal applications.

The **photo-disruptive effect** for capsulotomy or iridotomy requires high levels of energy, best achieved by the **Q-switched, pulsed mode**, to produce extremely short pulses of exceedingly high energy.

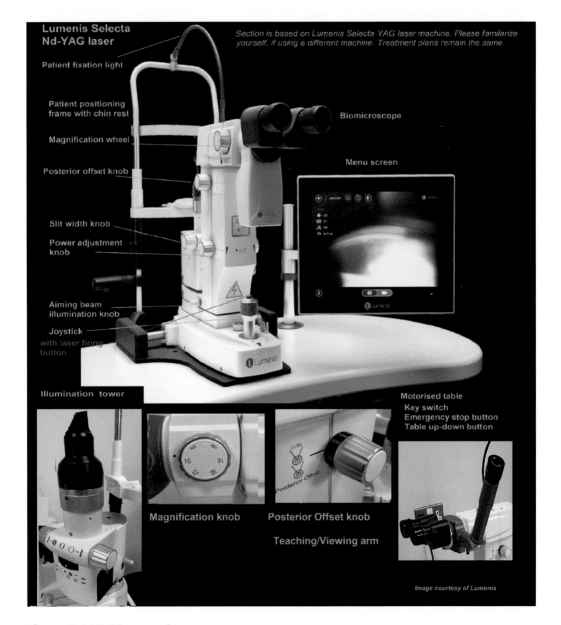

Figure 2.1 YAG laser machine.

DOI: 10.1201/9781003144304-3

33

2.1.1 Getting Started

- Switch on the mains and turn the ignition key. The **'power on' indicator light** comes on.
- Wait for the machine to boot up (perform a series of self-tests).
- **Select YAG or SLT from the LCD screen – home page.**
- The laser is on stand-by mode – safety shutter is closed, joystick button is disabled, and laser will not fire. **The laser will only activate when 'ready mode' is selected.**
- **Emergency off button de-energizes the system immediately, and the key ignition will not work if the emergency button has been activated.**

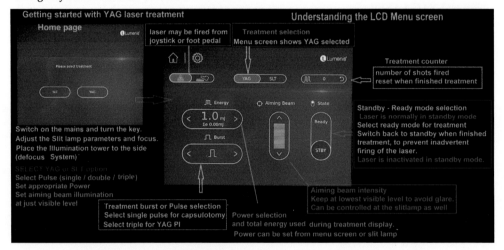

Figure 2.2 Getting started – understanding the LCD menu screen.

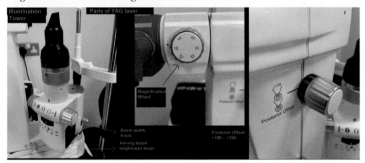

Figure 2.3 Parts of YAG laser.

Laser Settings

Adjust slit lamp – for table height, chin rest, eyepiece IPD, and refractive error.
- **Slit beam parameters – set slit at full height, medium width** (narrow slit sharpens focus or depth of perception but reduces FOV), and **just visible brightness** (to avoid glare).
- **Magnification** – low magnification (×6) for initial examination, high magnification (×16) for treatment.

Illumination tower – positioned appropriately (laser will not fire in the wrong position).
- **YAG option** – illumination tower is placed to the side (defocused system).
- **SLT option** – illumination tower is coaligned (parfocal system).

Aiming beam (diode) – set brightness at just visible level.

Inability to see the aiming beam may suggest:
- Suboptimal slit lamp focus. Refocus to improve view.
- Tilted contact lens that affects view of treatment area and aiming beam. Ensure CL is flat.
- Reduce slit lamp illumination. The aiming beam may be lost in the presence of extremely bright illumination.
- Increase aiming beam brightness slightly (very bright beam causes glare and trouble focusing on the treatment area precisely).

Power – can be altered from the slit lamp (clockwise to increase or anti-clockwise to decrease power) or from the LCD screen.
- **Screen displays selected power.**
Total energy = power used × number of shots; will display on the menu screen and can be reset back to zero at the end of treatment.

Shot selection
- The **burst mode** offers **single, double, or triple shots** for YAG treatment and is inactivated with SLT selection. The most appropriate options are:
  - **Single shot for capsulotomy**
  - **Triple shot for iridotomy.**
- Iridotomy can be done using single or double pulses but will require higher power and more shots to complete the procedure.

Laser defocus is related to treatment safety.
- **The aiming beam can be defocused up to +350 μm in front of the laser beam. Laser energy is delivered behind the aiming beam by the amount of defocus selected.**
- **Defocus is used to avoid IOL pitting.** If the opacified capsule is close to the IOL, laser focused on the capsule will inevitably hit the IOL. With appropriate defocus, the laser fired behind the PCO generates shockwaves that travel forwards to hit the capsule without damaging the IOL.
- **As shockwaves need to travel further forwards, slightly higher power may be needed, with a larger defocus.**
- **Set defocus at zero** – for LPI, anterior capsulotomy, clearance of SLM or IOL debris, and vitreolysis.
- **Set defocus at + 100–150 μm for regular posterior capsulotomy** (except in aphakes).
- **Increase defocus to +250–350 μm** – with adherent capsule (IOL pits despite initial defocus).

Select contact lens for treatment – used with topical anaesthetic and coupling lubricant.

Indications for YAG Laser
- **Posterior capsulotomy**
- **Anterior capsulotomy** – anterior capsular phimosis
- **Capsular block distension syndrome (CBDS)**
- **Peripheral iridotomy** – narrow angles, angle closure glaucoma, plateau iris
- Clearance of soft lens matter in visual axis after cataract surgery
- Clearance of pseudophakic inflammatory pupillary membrane, synechiae, and IOL debris in the visual axis
- **YAG vitreolysis** – for vitreous wick, with CMO, following complicated cataract surgery
- **SLT laser** for OHT and POAG
- Draining pre-macular subhyaloid haemorrhage
- Recurrent corneal erosion syndrome
- Cyclo-photoablation in refractory glaucoma
- Disruption of anterior hyaloid face in malignant glaucoma (rare)
- **Frequency doubled Nd-YAG used as photothermal lasers**

Laser Power Selection for Common YAG Procedures

Posterior capsulotomy	**1.0–1.5 mJ (depending on thickness of capsule).** **Most posterior capsulotomy can be done with 1–1.2 mJ power.**
Anterior capsulotomy	**1.0–2.0 mJ, depending on thickness of the anterior capsular phimosis (phimosed edge may be thicker).**
Clearance of pupillary membrane	**1.0-1.2 mJ is usually adequate for most cases. Very thick membranes need slightly higher power.**
Clearance of IOL deposits	**0.6–0.8 mJ (use extremely low power).**
Clearance of SLM	**1.5–2.5 mJ (based on thickness of soft lens matter).**
YAG iridotomy, plateau iris	**1.5 mJ ×3 pulse = 4.5 mJ for thin iris.** **3 mJ × 3 shot = 9 mJ for thick iris.** **Most PI can be done using 4.5–7.5 mJ. Select power based on iris thickness. Do not start with low power on a thick iris.**
YAG vitreolysis	**2–4 mJ (unpigmented vitreous needs higher power).**
SLT	**0.7–1.2 mJ**
YAG hyaloidotomy	**4–5 mJ, titrate up to get perforation**
RES	**0.3–0.6 mJ (low power) in recurrent erosion syndrome**

2.2 YAG LASER POSTERIOR CAPSULOTOMY

Posterior capsular opacification is the commonest late complication of cataract surgery, causing blurred vision, glare, reduced contrast sensitivity, and monocular diplopia. A unilateral PCO can reduce binocularity and stereopsis, and affect QoL.

Nd-YAG capsulotomy is a safe and effective treatment with success rates of 85–95% and should be considered for visually symptomatic patients.

Previous incidence of PCO was approximately 20% at 2 years and 30% at 5 years. Advances in surgical techniques, IOL materials, and designs have reduced and delayed PCO rates but not eliminated it entirely. It still poses a significant problem, in adults, 5–10 years after cataract surgery (15–30%), with much higher incidence in infants and children (100% within 2 years).

YAG capsulotomy involves clearing the visual axis by creating a central opening in the opacified posterior capsule. Improvement in acuity, glare, and contrast sensitivity are important outcome measures for patients.

2.2.1 Pathophysiology of Posterior Capsular Opacification

The lens capsule has 2 zones of lens epithelial cells, central LEC (anterior and posterior capsule), and equatorial LEC (lens bow).

There is proliferation, migration, and epithelial-mesenchymal transformation (EMT) of residual LEC, left in the capsular bag after cataract surgery, causing pseudo-fibrous metaplasia. The metaplastic myofibroblast produces fibrin and collagen causing PCO.

Mesenchymal changes cause fibrotic contractions, inducing wrinkles on the posterior capsule, causing glare, trouble with night driving, annoying streaks, and starburst light effects, due to the capsular folds acting as cylindrical lenses (**Maddox rod effect**).

Equatorial bow LECs are important in formation of **Elshnig's pearls** (aberrant attempt of LEC to form new lens fibres), which are thicker and more visually debilitating. Sometimes, pearls spread in a circular fashion along the edge of a small anterior capsulorhexis, causing a **Soemmerring's ring (capsular phimosis)**.

This process is **influenced by multiple growth factors, cytokines, and extracellular matrix proteins** (*Transforming growth factor β (TGF-β), fibroblast growth factor2 (FGF-2) hepatocyte growth factor, interleukins 1 and 6 (IL-1 and IL-6), and epithelial growth factor*).

Pre-existing ocular inflammatory diseases or inflammation from surgical complications enhance fibrosis, appearing as whitish-grey bands or plaques, thicker at the IOL edges, months to years after surgery. Fibrosis presenting soon after surgery usually represents SLM remnants, left behind during surgery.

Good cortical clean-up and PC polishing during cataract surgery reduces PCO incidence, but over-aggressive capsular polishing is neither possible nor advisable, due to the risk of PCR (PC rupture), and some LECs are necessary for capsular bag integrity, to support and stabilize the IOL post-operatively.

New research, exploring methods to modulate LECs, prevent fibrosis, and maintain bag integrity will become important, with the advent of new accommodating IOLs that rely on an intact posterior capsule.

2.2.2 Posterior Capsular Opacification in Paediatric Patients

PCO occurs in 40–100% of children and young adults after cataract surgery, due to more marked inflammatory and healing responses to

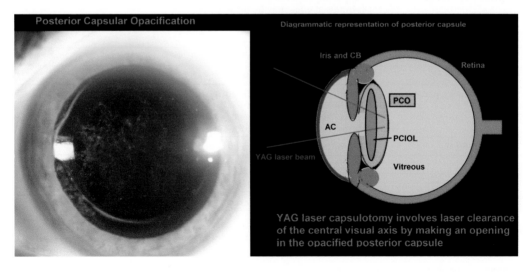

Figure 2.4 PCO.

a surgical insult. Recent advances in paediatric cataract surgery, with posterior continuous curvilinear capsulorhexis and anterior vitrectomy, have reduced the incidence.

- PCO is **potentially sight threatening** in children, due to **higher incidence rate, quicker onset, denser opacification, and greater amblyogenic effect on vision.**

- **Primary posterior capsulotomy with anterior vitrectomy (during cataract surgery), is the preferred treatment to prevent PCO.**

- If this has not been done, a YAG capsulotomy may be performed in older children.

PCO development is influenced by age, pre-existing inflammation, and history of trauma. Cataract surgery can be difficult in such patients, with increased risk of retained SLM, iris adhesions, capsular pigment migration, and persistent inflammation.

Factors That Influence PCO Formation
Patient-Related Factors
Age – common in young patients, infants, and children. **Systemic and ocular diseases** – PXF syndrome, myotonic dystrophy, chronic uveitis, retinitis pigmentosa, traumatic cataract, and high myopia (likely due difficult surgery). Diabetics have a lower incidence but tend to have thicker PCO.
Surgery-Related Factors
Higher PCO rates – poor surgical technique and intraoperative complications, too small or large capsulorhexis, incomplete hydro-dissection, cortical/SLM remnants, excessive surgical manipulation, PCR, IO silicone oil, ECCE, all increase PCO rate. **Lower PCO rates** – good surgical techniques (reduces postoperative inflammation). CCC slightly smaller than IOL optic (edge of anterior capsule is over the IOL optic, and not in contact with PC), good hydro-dissection, sealed capsule irrigation system, good I&A, and cortical clean-up (removal of all regenerative and viscoelastic materials), in the bag IOL fixation and good PC polish, all reduce the risk.
IOL-Related Factors (Material and Design)
Higher PCO rates – hydrophilic IOL, cheap poor-quality lens, broad haptic-optic junction, single-piece IOL, all support LEC adhesion, migration, and proliferation. **Hydrogel IOLs are associated with the highest rate of PCO.** **Lower PCO rates** – lens material – hydrophobic IOLs like silicone, acrylic IOL. **Lens modifications** – posterior IOL surface convexity, posterior angulation of haptic, larger IOL optic, thicker IOL, slim haptic-optic junction, sharp square truncated IOL edge (less space between PC and IOL optic for LEC migration). **IOL surface coating** (heparin, Teflon, titanium, carbon) inhibits LEC migration and protein adhesion.

2.2.3 Types of Capsular Opacification

PCO classification is based on appearance and severity (mild, moderate, severe)

Membranous/Fibrous PCO • Caused by central LEC changes, with varying degrees of folds, wrinkles, and fibrosis. • Symptoms range from glare to visual loss. • Capsulotomy requires lower power and fewer shots. • Well-focused shots cause splits in the posterior capsule, which connect to complete the procedure with less inflammation.	**Membranous / Fibrous PCO** 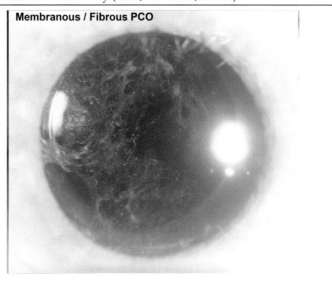
	Figure 2.5 Membranous PCO.

Pearl Type PCO
- Caused by equatorial LEC metaplasia, thick, irregular PCO, likely to affect vision.
- Anterior migration of pearls causes anterior capsular phimosis and capsular distention syndrome.
- Needs higher laser power and more shots to complete capsulotomy.
- Laser causes punch holes rather than splits in thick areas with a greater inflammatory response.

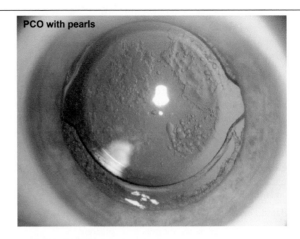

Figure 2.6 PCO with pearls.

Mixed PCO (fibrosis + pearls)
- Commonest presentation.
- Choosing thin areas within the pearls makes treatment easier.
- AC inflammation settles downward and may obscure the view, affecting completion.
- With thick pearls, it is advisable to start treatment inferiorly and then move upwards.
- Severe inflammation affecting visibility may require capsulotomy to be deferred until the inflammation has settled with treatment.

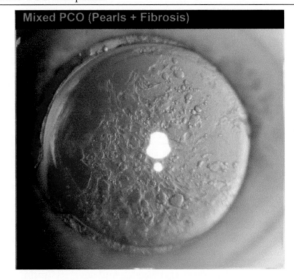

Figure 2.7 Mixed PCO.

Posterior Capsular Plaque
- Usually associated with a dense PSCLO (posterior subcapsular lenticular opacity).
- Should be removed intraoperatively with good I&A and capsular polishing.
- Adherent plaques have a high risk of PCR with polishing, and YAG capsulotomy at 3–6 months may be the safer option. Cautious treatment is advised (minimum power and shots) as remaining capsule is thin and clear.

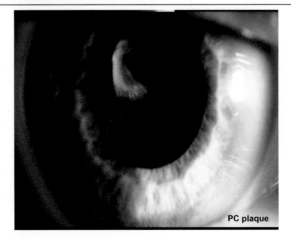

Figure 2.8 PC plaque.

Capsular Folds/Wrinkles
- Capsule is not opacified, but presence of capsular folds can be visually disabling due to Maddox rod effect.
- With severe symptoms, a cautious YAG capsulotomy can be done after careful patient counselling.

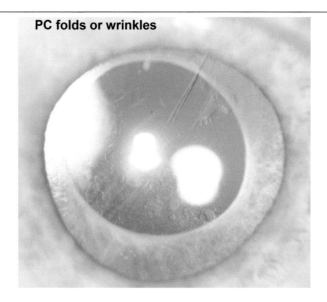

PC folds or wrinkles

Figure 2.9 PCO folds.

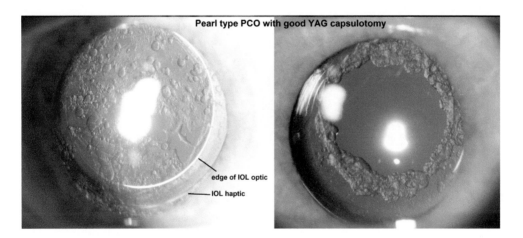

Pearl type PCO with good YAG capsulotomy

edge of IOL optic

IOL haptic

Figure 2.10 Good YAG capsulotomy.

2.2.4 How Does YAG Laser Work?

Capsulotomy is done using **the Q-switched Nd-YAG laser (wavelength 1064 nm), in the photo-disruptor mode.** This delivers a high level of energy in a short pulse, at the target area, ionizing cells and surrounding fluid to create a plasma bubble, which expands and collapses, generating forward moving acoustic shockwaves that disrupt nearby tissues (posterior capsule, IOL) – **photomechanical effect**.

- **Posterior offset (+100–350 μm)** is used to prevent IOL pitting.

- Contact lens use helps stabilize the eye, magnify the view, improve focus, and reduce treatment power needed. A contact lens makes the procedure safer by increasing the cone angle from 16° to 24°.

2.2.5 YAG Capsulotomy

PCO can occur from the immediate postoperative period to years after cataract surgery. In visually symptomatic patients, treatment is essential but is best avoided immediately after cataract surgery.

Capsulotomy is not advisable within 3 months of cataract surgery due to increased risk of complications – CMO, VMT, uveitis, RD.

Contraindications for YAG Capsulotomy	
Relative contraindications	Absolute contraindication
Capsulotomy can be done cautiously, with low power, minimal shots, small opening, and informed consent of higher risks. Defer procedure if possible. • Previous retinal tears or detachment. • High myopes. • Recurrent or active uveitis – *risk of flare up (treat under steroid cover).* • Pre-existing CMO. • 3–6 months after cataract surgery. • Uncontrolled glaucoma. • Small, non-dilating pupil. • Inability to fixate eyes. • Non-co-operative patients.	• Corneal opacification, oedema, or dystrophy (poor view of aiming beam and capsule, degradation of laser beam prevents reliable, predictable photo-disruption, hazy cornea scatters laser light, leading to increased risk of corneal burns). • **Within 6–8 weeks following cataract surgery**, due to higher risks of complications especially CMO and RD. • Eyes with poor visual potential.

2.2.6 YAG Capsulotomy Techniques – Two Main Techniques

Cruciate Pattern

- Creates a cross pattern of laser shots – uses fewer shots and less energy.
- Resultant four triangular capsular flaps (still attached peripherally) fold back and retract out of the visual axis.

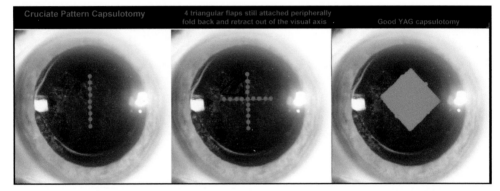

Figure 2.11 Cruciate YAG capsulotomy.

- **Benefits** – fewer shots used, avoids creation of free-floating capsular fragments, lowers risk of floaters and retinal detachment.
- **Risks** – flaps may fold back into the visual axis, higher risk of IOL pitting in the visual axis as shots cross the central area (avoided by good focusing).
- Central pits affect vision significantly, making this technique less popular.

Circular Pattern (Can Opener Capsulotomy)

Can opener capsulotomy is preferred by most users as it avoids the central visual axis but takes a little more energy and time to complete. Create a 'circular pattern' of laser shots for a round PC opening. A large central fragment can be broken up with a few shots to allow quick absorption and clearance.

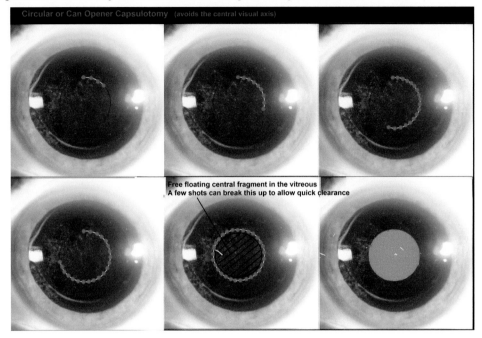

Circular or Can Opener Capsulotomy (avoids the central visual axis)

Free floating central fragment in the vitreous
A few shots can break this up to allow quick clearance

Figure 2.12 Can opener YAG capsulotomy.

- **Benefit** – avoids central optical zone, reducing risk of central IOL pits. Peripheral pits do not affect vision significantly.
- **Risks** – more shots required, creation of a free-floating capsular fragment in the vitreous (floaters in vision) and slightly higher risk of RD.

2.2.7 Treatment Procedure

Examine patients prior to procedure, to ensure safe treatment, with no surprises. Informed consent is taken after risks and benefits have been explained clearly.

The aim is to improve vision and reduce glare and other visual problems.

Patient examination – document:
- **BCVA (best corrected visual acuity)**, IOP, coexisting ocular/systemic problems (may affect procedure/outcomes).
- **Type/thickness of capsule.**
- **Presence of eccentric pupil.**
- **Poor patient co-operation** – poor placement at slit lamp, communication problems, nystagmus, tremor, difficult patients.

- **Pupils can be eccentric or dilate eccentrically. Inattention may result in a decentred capsulotomy.**
- **Do not dilate patients with eccentric pupil. Document the visual axis centred to the eccentric pupil so that the capsulotomy can be located appropriately.**

Pre-treatment Work-up
- A small pupil results in a small capsulotomy, with visual problems from edge effect of the capsular remnant. It is therefore advisable to dilate BE with **tropicamide 1%** to facilitate capsular visualization (except with eccentric pupil).
- **It is best to have mid-dilated pupils**. A widely dilated pupil may result in a larger than desired capsulotomy, which can destabilize the IOL.
- Apraclonidine (or other IOP drops) instilled pre- and post-treatment prevents an IOP spike.

- **Use Abraham's Capsulotomy CL with topical anaesthesia and coupling lubricant.**
- Ensure patient is comfortable, keep their head still, and maintain steady fixation during treatment. Seek assistance with difficult, nervous, or unco-operative patients.

YAG Laser Machine

- Switch the laser on. Select YAG option from home page.
- Place **illumination tower appropriately** to the side (defocus system).
- **Set power at 1.0–1.5mJ** based on capsule thickness. Select **single pulse.**

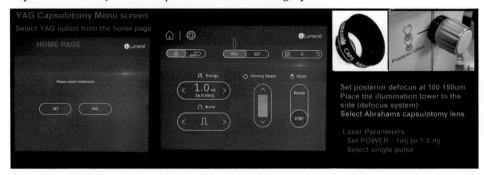

Figure 2.13 YAG capsulotomy menu page.

Laser Defocus (Posterior Offset)
- **Set + 100–150 μm posterior offset. Alter defocus, based on reaction.**
- Constant pitting of IOL – increase defocus.
- Disturbance of vitreous without touching the capsule – reduce defocus.
- With a **larger defocus, laser energy required will be slightly higher.**
- **Aphakic eyes with PCO do not need defocus, as there is no IOL to pit. The focus can be set directly on the posterior capsule** (defocus=0).

- **Select ready** when both patient and doctor ready.
- **YAG laser will show 2 red lights – aiming beam** (4 in some machines).
- **Align the 2 aiming beams to a sharp single spot on the capsule and fire.**
- **Good focus is vital. Treatment in the right plane results in a capsular split. Well positioned shots cause splits to connect and complete the treatment.**

Aiming Beam
You get multiple reflections of the red aiming beam – from the cornea, IOL, and capsule. Ensure you are focused on the capsule, the posterior-most red light seen. If in doubt, pull slit lamp back and gradually go in to refocus on the capsule. You will appreciate multiple reflections by turning down the slit-lamp illumination. The corneal reflection is too far forwards and easy to ignore. The IOL reflection is just ahead of the PCO reflection and tends to be brighter but fuzzy and can interfere with viewing the PCO aiming beam. Picking the appropriate aiming beam becomes easy with practice.

Procedure
Starting at 12 o'clock, move sequentially and clockwise placing shots at regular intervals to connect splits. If you get punch holes rather than splits, it suggests poor focus, a thicker capsule, or low power selection. Improve your focus first, then increase the power slightly if needed.

YAG Laser Capsulotomy Parameters – Can Opener Technique
Number of shots: 20–40 × Power 1–1.5 mJ × defocus 100–150 μm × single shot × Abraham's capsulotomy lens. (Complete treatment with least power and number of shots.)
Make a medium sized capsular opening: 3–5 mm diameter.
Do not make capsulotomy larger than the IOL optic (usually 6 mm) – it may destabilize the IOL, causing vitreous prolapse, with associated problems of inflammation, raised IOP, VMT, and CMO.

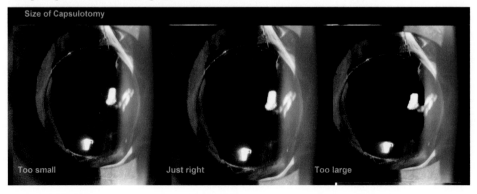

Figure 2.14 Size of capsulotomy.

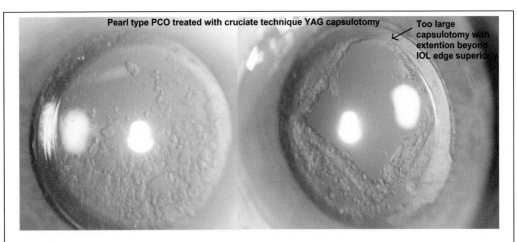

Figure 2.15 PCO treated with large YAG capsulotomy.

Post Laser Treatment
- Topical apraclonidine or other glaucoma drops prevent an IOP spike.
- Steroid drops for a week settle post laser inflammation.
- If unsure about completion of capsulotomy, review and complete in 2 weeks.
- Most patients are discharged with warning signs of PVD/retinal detachment, advising urgent attention if necessary.
- Co-existing ocular pathology should be followed up appropriately in the eye clinic.
- Patients are advised to see their optician in 4–6 weeks for refraction and glasses.

2.2.8 Size of the Posterior Capsulotomy

Although capsulotomy can be done with an undilated pupil, it results in a small opening. Physiological mydriasis exposes the edges of the opacified capsule causing glare and visual problems in scotopic conditions, such as driving at night.

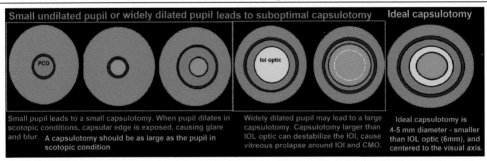

Figure 2.16 Pupil size and capsulotomy.

An ideal capsulotomy should be as large as the pupil in scotopic conditions.

- A **smaller opening is preferred in patients at high risk of retinal detachment** (low laser energy, reduce vitreous disturbance).
- A **slightly larger capsulotomy is preferred in diabetic patients**, to aid fundal view for future photothermal treatment.

- **If pupil is mid-dilated, follow pupillary edge to get a good capsulotomy**.
- With widely dilated pupils, do not follow the pupil edge, as you end up with a large capsulotomy, requiring more shots with increased risk of complications.
- Capsulotomy > IOL optic size is associated with more complications.

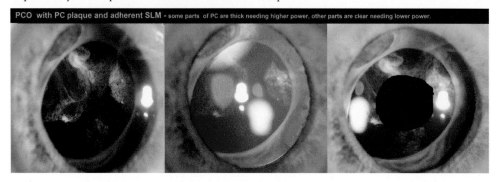

PCO with PC plaque and adherent SLM - some parts of PC are thick needing higher power, other parts are clear needing lower power.

Figure 2.17 PCO with plaque treated with capsulotomy.

2.2.9 YAG Capsulotomy with Eccentric Pupil

- It is important to check for the presence of an eccentric pupil before dilation.
- Dilating an eccentric pupil may cause loss of centration of the functional visual axis and lead to inappropriate placement of capsulotomy, causing ongoing visual problems with glare and blurred vision from the edge of the remaining capsule in the visual axis.
- **Do not dilate an eccentric pupil, and perform the capsulotomy centred to the eccentric pupil.**

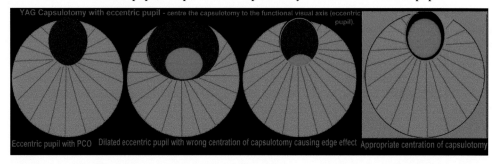

YAG Capsulotomy with eccentric pupil - centre the capsulotomy to the functional visual axis (eccentric pupil).

Eccentric pupil with PCO   Dilated eccentric pupil with wrong centration of capsulotomy causing edge effect   Appropriate centration of capsulotomy

Figure 2.18 YAG capsulotomy with eccentric pupil.

2.2.10 Complications of YAG Capsulotomy

YAG capsulotomy is an effective treatment, but not without risks, especially with the presence of a cloudy cornea, small, or eccentric pupil, and high degree of astigmatism, with difficulty in focusing, leading to excessive energy use, laser scattering and higher risk of complications.

The risk of complications increases with use of higher power and number of shots.

Visual problems	• Loss of vision, glare, nyctalopia, negative dysphotopsia (darkening of vision), positive dysphotopsia (dazzling, disabling light), and floaters. The symptoms may be related to IOL pits, IOL tilt/movement after the procedure.
CL-related problem	• Corneal injury, abrasion, erosions, conjunctivitis (poor technique and contact lens hygiene).
Cornea *(avoid eye makeup on treatment day)*	• Corneal oedema, endothelial cell loss, burns due to poor focus. • Corneal perforation from inadvertent laser absorption by pigment trapped between the eye and contact lens (mascara, eyelash).

Iris	• Iris haemorrhage, hyphema, and transient iritis can occur if lasering close to pupillary margin (resolves with steroids).
Exacerbation of localized endophthalmitis	• Propionibacterium acnes endophthalmitis can occur following treatment. The capsulotomy is presumed to allow organisms sequestered within the bag to reach the vitreous and cause a low grade endophthalmitis.
IOL **Pitting of IOL** **(15–33%)**	• **Common with hazy view, poor focusing, poor laser technique, and silicon lens (less with acrylic lens). Usually not visually disabling, but severe pitting causes glare, image degradation, and may need IOL removal.** • **IOL subluxation or displacement – with over-sized capsulotomy. IOL dislocation into the vitreous has been reported.** • **A backward movement of the IOL can occur soon after a capsulotomy, causing a hyperopic refractive shift. It is therefore advisable to defer a visit to the optician for 3–4 weeks following the procedure.**
Vitreous	Disruption of posterior hyaloid face may cause vitreous prolapse into the AC, corneal oedema from vitreo-corneal touch, rise in IOP, uveitis, vitritis, VMT with CMO, and vitreous haemorrhage.
IOP **Transient rise in IOP is the commonest complication after posterior capsulotomy (15–30% cases)** Usually resolves with treatment	High IOP can be due to reduced outflow from pupil block, inflammatory debris or vitreous prolapse blocking TM, aqueous misdirection, possible steroid response, and TM damage from photo-disruptive shockwaves (explains link with use of higher energy). IOP tends to be higher and more persistent, requiring treatment in patients with pre-existing glaucoma, aphakia, previous ECCE without a surgical PI, myopes, and pre-existing VR diseases. **High IOP is greater with the use of higher laser power (>1.5 mJ), excessive shots, or a larger capsulotomy.** • Care must be taken in trabeculectomy patients, as capsulotomy may have a negative impact on the filtering bleb, causing loss of IOP control (related to vitreous obstruction of sclerostomy).
Macular problems	• Macular problems (CMO, ERM, VMT, macular hole) can occur (0.5–2.5%) due to disturbance of vitreous, VMT, and release of inflammatory mediators. **CMO is more common with capsulotomy within 6/12 of cataract surgery.**
Retina *Extreme care in high-risk patient, use lower energy and reduced number of shots to prevent RD.*	• Retinal haemorrhage, tears, detachment can occur after capsulotomy (common in men with high myopia). **Retinal detachment rate is 0.1–3.6%, especially if treatment was done soon after cataract surgery.** • Cataract surgery itself is a risk for RD (0.8–1%), and YAG capsulotomy increases the risk further (1.6–1.9%). • The risk of RD is higher with axial myopia, pre-existing VR pathology, PCR, previous history of RD, and lattice degeneration. • **AVOID capsulotomy within 6 months of surgery.**

Failure to improve vision after treatment is often due to pre-existing ocular diseases

2.2.11 IOL Pitting

IOL pitting is an undesirable complication of YAG capsulotomy and usually occurs due to poor technique. One to 2 peripheral pits may be acceptable and do not affect vision significantly, but multiple pits, or central pits, can be visually disabling.

Good practice with laser treatment is essential to reduce the risk of IOL pits.
- **Sharp focus on the capsule is vital**.
- **Always use a contact lens**. It increases the cone angle and reduces risk of damage to surrounding tissues.
- **Ensure CL is flat on the eye.** CL tilt affects the view, introduces air bubbles, and constant CL manipulation affects corneal clarity, making the procedure difficult.
- **Set defocus +100–150** (*aiming beam is focused on the capsule – laser is delivered 100–150 μm behind the capsule, causing shockwaves to disrupt the capsule, without affecting the IOL*).
- If pits still occur, increase defocus to +250 to +350. Power needs to be increased slightly with higher defocus, as shockwaves need to travel further forwards.
- **Always do capsulotomy in a planned manner.**
  - **Use the least power** needed.
  - **DO NOT RUSH treatment** (only fire when aiming beams are perfectly aligned).
  - Start mid-peripherally at 12 o'clock, and move clockwise, in a curvilinear fashion to create a flap – this pushes the remaining capsule away from the IOL.
  - If an IOL pit affects your view, move to the next quadrant – once you create a capsular flap, you can come back and treat the affected area.
  - Avoid retreating (multiple shots) the same area.
  - **Anticipate need for help** – patients with head tremors, neck stiffness, dementia, confusion, language barrier, poor co-operation, anxious, young, or very elderly patients, and those with pre-existing ocular conditions.
- If IOL pits occur consistently, with multiple users – check slit lamp eyepiece focus, and ensure that slit lamp is calibrated and serviced.
- **Consider an opacified IOL** – stop treatment if you get constant IOL pits – it may be an adherent capsule, or an opacified IOL. Seek senior advice. In the presence of an opacified IOL, an intact PC will aid IOL exchange.

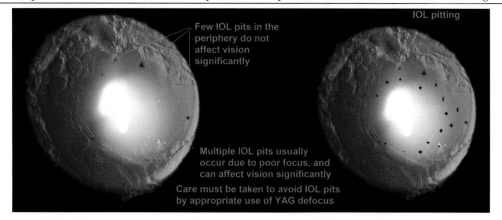

Figure 2.19 IOL pitting.

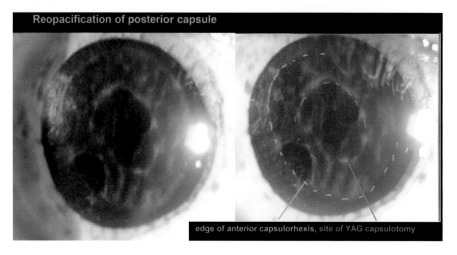

Figure 2.20 Re-opacification of PC.

2.2.12 Newer Concepts in Posterior Capsulotomy

- **Dodick phacolysis** – thorough removal of cortical material from capsule equator while keeping anterior capsular rim LEC intact, to preserve capsular integrity.

- **Femtolaser** – performs precise capsulorhexis and cataract surgery (reduces PCO).

- **Zepto capsulotomy device** – uses laser to remove the laminin layer of the posterior capsule, shown to reduce PCO formation.

- **Primary posterior laser capsulotomy (PPLC)** – Some surgeons advocate opening the posterior capsule during cataract surgery using femtolaser after IOL implantation.

2.2.13 Re-opacification of Posterior Capsule

True re-opacification is rare and more likely due to development of an inflammatory pupillary membrane. Patients may develop re-opacification, in presence of iritis with a small stuck down pupil, as it stimulates formation of an inflammatory pupillary membrane, or migration of pearls from the capsulotomy edge can close a small capsular opening.

2.2.14 IOL Opacification/Calcification

IOL calcification is a rare occurrence, often misdiagnosed as posterior capsular opacification, presenting as surface glistening, calcification, or snowflake degeneration, which cannot be removed by laser. They should not be confused with inflammatory IOL deposits after cataract surgery, which clear with anti-inflammatory drops and laser treatment.

It is more common with hydrophilic acrylic lenses, silicone lenses, and memory lenses, and can affect the lens surface, sub-surface, or intra-lens material. There is documented association with chronic inflammatory eye diseases, asteroid hyalosis, and VR surgery.

PMMA lenses can show progressive snowflake degeneration affecting the central visual axis, from long-term exposure to UV light (lens periphery is protected by the iris and not affected). Acrylic lenses may show fluid-filled microvacuoles (glistening).

IOL opacification is often misdiagnosed as PCO

Often misdiagnosed as PCO, and attempted YAG capsulotomy leads to constant IOL pitting, despite maximum defocus, worsening visual symptoms.

- A high index of suspicion, and detailed slit lamp examination under higher magnification is necessary for diagnosis.
- If IOL opacification is severe, the view may be hazy and diagnosis difficult.
- If in doubt, seek a second opinion before performing any procedure.

These patients often require IOL exchange and need to have an intact capsule.
Avoid performing a YAG capsulotomy in these patients. YAG capsulotomy makes IOL exchange more difficult, with higher risk of surgical and post-surgical complications, with increased ocular morbidity

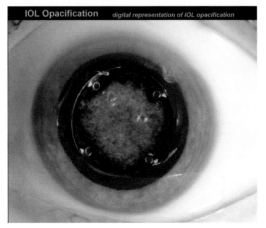

IOL Opacification   *digital representation of IOL opacification*

Figure 2.21 IOL opacification.

2.3 CAPSULAR BLOCK DISTENSION SYNDROME

CBDS is a rare complication of cataract surgery (0.73%), occurring weeks, months, or years later, and usually associated with:

- Small continuous curvilinear capsulorhexis (CCC)

- PCIOL especially with four haptics

- Axial length >25 mm

- leaving viscoelastic material and SLM in the bag

- anterior capsular phimosis.

2.3.1 Pathophysiology of CBDS

CBDS occurs due to accumulation of fluid, retained lens matter, and viscoelastic debris between the PCIOL and posterior capsule, leading to distension of the capsular bag and anterior displacement of IOL. The trapped fluid becomes turbid, causing a refractive shift (commonly myopic, occasionally hyperopic) and decreased vision.

Presentation is variable with intraoperative, early, or late postoperative onset.

Intraoperative CBDS
- Due to high irrigation pressure during hydro-dissection, in the presence of a small capsulorhexis. The bag is distended with clear fluid and associated with increased risk of posterior capsular rupture.

Early Postoperative CBDS
- Due to incomplete removal of viscoelastic material during surgery (non-cellular, inflammatory changes), causing anterior displacement of IOL, shallowing of AC, IOP elevation, and a myopic shift.

Late Postoperative CBDS
- Associated with LEC remnants, undergoing EMT with fibrosis and phimosis of the anterior capsule (Soemmerring ring). The fluid is turbid (sign of chronicity). Changes are cellular and fibrotic.

Most cases are associated with:
- Small capsulorhexis (<5 mm), adherent to IOL.
- **Turbid fluid (varying from clear to milky) between IOL and PC, causing a retro-lenticular pseudo-hypopyon.**
- Some cases have associated IOL glistening or opacification.
- The PC may be clear or opacified but may be difficult to see through the turbid fluid.

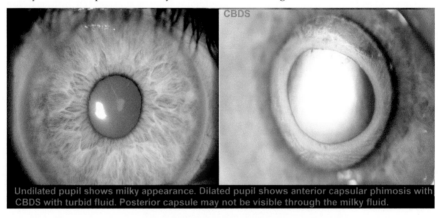

Undilated pupil shows milky appearance. Dilated pupil shows anterior capsular phimosis with CBDS with turbid fluid. Posterior capsule may not be visible through the milky fluid.

Figure 2.22 CBDS.

Ideally, CBDS should be diagnosed in clinic (pre-laser).

2.3.1.1 CBDS Presentation

- Blurred vision
- Media opacity
- Myopic refractive shift
- Anterior capsule phimosis
- Retro-lenticular hypopyon
- Shallowing of AC
- Forward bowing of iris
- Narrow angles with occasional rise in IOP.
- Forward movement of IOL, may cause pupil block glaucoma (rare).
- Distended capsular bag with posterior capsule way behind the IOL (may not be visible with turbid fluid.
- PCO (may be absent in early CBDS)
- Small anterior capsulorhexis (4mm) with IOL optic and anterior capsular rim adhesions.
- Confirmed with **AS-OCT, Pentacam, or anterior UBM.**

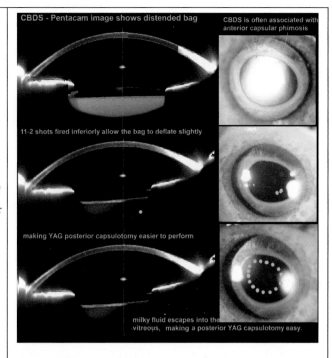

Figure 2.23 CBDS – Pentacam.

Difficulty in viewing capsule, turbid, milky white fluid in the bag, and trouble performing capsulotomy are suggestive of CBDS during laser treatment.
- **Laser shots disturb the bag fluid, without causing a capsular split or punch hole, normally seen with a capsulotomy.**

- Rarely, a late presentation of CBDS causes or mimics Propionibacterium acnes endophthalmitis, with pain, irritation, redness, and low-grade inflammation in the AC. A capsulotomy may release virulent organisms sequestered in the distended bag.
- If P. acnes endophthalmitis is suspected (CBDS, with excessive inflammation) prior to laser treatment, then a pars plana vitrectomy, removal of debris, and total capsulotomy may be necessary.

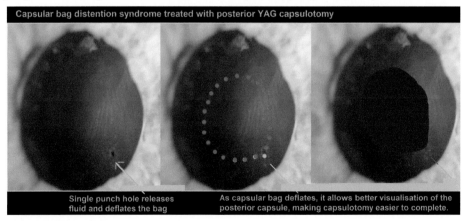

Figure 2.24 CBDS treatment.

Treatment of CBDS is YAG posterior capsulotomy.
2–30 shots × single pulse × 1.5–2 mJ power × 0 defocus × Abraham's lens.
Start with 2–3 shots inferiorly.

- **The posterior capsule is further back, and you need to go in with the slit lamp to focus on it.** Once focused, the procedure is like a standard posterior capsulotomy.
  Make 1–2 punch holes, inferiorly on the capsule (gravity allows some of the milky fluid to drain into the vitreous, reducing the distention, making completion of capsulotomy easier).
- **If PC is not visible, consider doing an anterior capsulotomy with 4–6 releasing incisions. This relieves blockage and allows the turbid fluid to drain into the AC.**
- **Posterior capsulotomy if still required can be completed at a second session a few weeks later. If the PC is not opacified, this may not be necessary.**

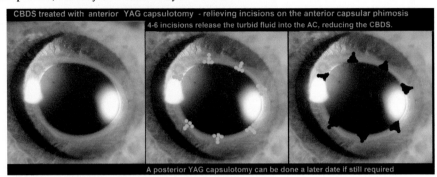

Figure 2.25 CBDS treated with anterior YAG capsulotomy.

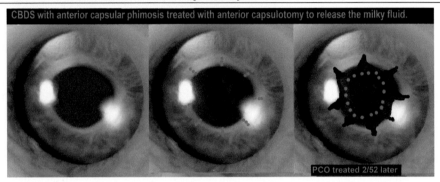

Figure 2.26 CBDS with anterior and posterior YAG capsulotomy.

- Pre- and post-treatment apraclonidine prevents an IOP spike, related to excessive inflammation.
- Persistent high IOP an hour later may require a course of topical glaucoma drops.
- **Intensive steroids are required to suppress excessive inflammation.**
- Review in 4–6 weeks to ensure inflammation has settled and capsulotomy is complete.
  Patients will have **a significant refractive shift following treatment** and will need to see their optician in 6 weeks.

2.4 ANTERIOR CAPSULOTOMY

Capsular contraction syndrome (CCS)

(Soemmerring ring) represents an exaggerated response of metaplastic lens epithelial cells (LEC), causing anterior capsular phimosis, usually within 2–3 months after cataract surgery.

- Common with silicon IOLs in patients with pseudo-exfoliation syndrome, diabetic retinopathy, uveitis, retinitis pigmentosa, and myotonic dystrophy.
- The phimosis can be severe enough to **affect visual axis, displace IOL**, and cause **zonular rupture and capsular block distention syndrome (CBDS)**

- Preventive measures include performing a larger capsulorhexis (diameter 5–6mm), good hydro-dissection, eliminating all SLM during irrigation and aspiration through capsular polishing, and avoiding, silicone IOLs.

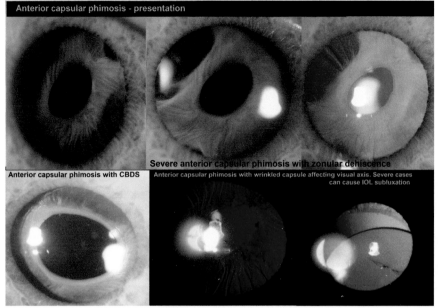

Figure 2.27 Anterior capsular phimosis presentation.

Anterior Capsulotomy
- Pre- and post-treatment plans are similar to posterior capsulotomy.
- YAG capsulotomy is done on the phimosed edge to release scarring. With thick phimosis, laser power may need to be increased slightly.
- Place between four and ten releasing radial laser incisions (3–5 shots per radial incision) equidistantly to open up the phimosis.
- 20–40 shots × 1.5-2.5 mJ power × single pulse × Abraham's lens × defocus 0.

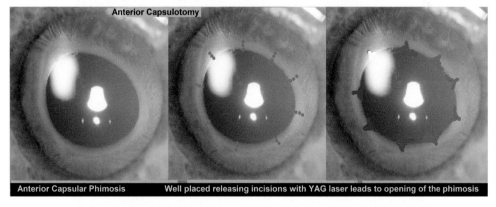

Figure 2.28 Anterior capsulotomy – 1.

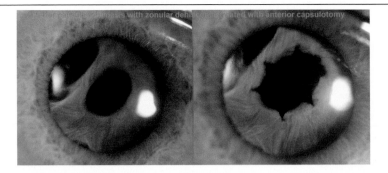

Figure 2.29 Anterior capsulotomy – 2.

Complications of laser – IOL displacement, IOP spike, uveitis, iris trauma, and hyphema. Associated irido-capsular adhesion, posterior synechiae, and retained SLM may need treatment.

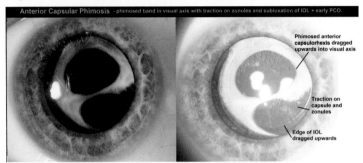

Figure 2.30 Anterior capsular phimosis – 1.

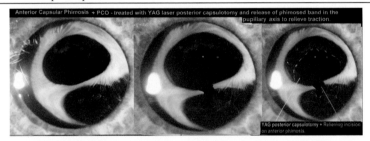

Figure 2.31 Anterior capsular phimosis – treated.

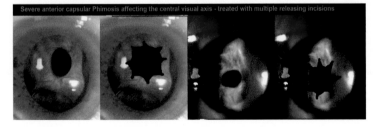

Figure 2.32 Severe anterior capsular phimosis.

2.5 INFLAMMATORY PUPILLARY MEMBRANE AND SYNECHIOLYSIS IN PSEUDOPHAKES

Inflammatory pupillary membrane occurs due to disruption of blood aqueous barrier, allowing fibrin, plasma proteins, and inflammatory cells to collect on the IOL surface and form a pupillary membrane, causing glare and blurred vision with poor fundal view.

Conditions that disrupt blood aqueous barrier causing increased vascular permeability are more likely to cause inflammatory membranes. A small stuck-down pupil promotes LEC migration across the pupil, making the membrane thicker.
- Pseudo exfoliation syndrome.
- Microangiopathy – diabetic retinopathy.
- Glaucoma patients on pilocarpine, longstanding miosis.
- Chronic uveitis.
- Difficult cataract surgery with retained SLM, persistent post-op inflammation.

Pseudophakes with an inflammatory pupillary membrane or localized synechiae due to recurrent chronic uveitis can be treated cautiously with YAG laser, in an eye with good visual potential.
Early treatment is key; chronic extensive synechiae are unlikely to benefit.
Early and localized synechiae may be broken by aggressive pupillary dilatation and active treatment of their uveitis with intensive steroids.

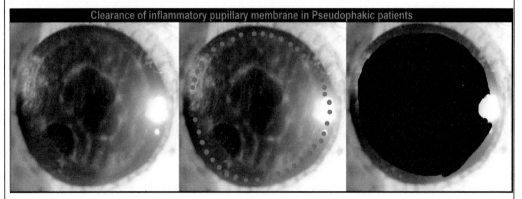

Figure 2.33 YAG clearance of inflammatory pupillary membrane.

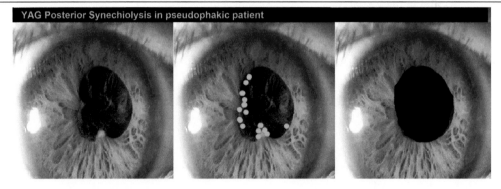

Figure 2.34 YAG posterior synechiolysis.

Laser treatment will flare up uveitis and is not advisable with active inflammation.
- **With chronic inflammatory disease, the pupillary membrane or synechiae may recur despite treatment.** Rarely, a hyphema may occur from iris trauma. Patients must be warned of risk of flare-up and possible failure of treatment.
- **Treat during a stable phase, early in the disease spectrum (early and few synechiae), under intensive and prolonged steroid cover.**

Laser treatment for inflammatory membrane and synechiae in pseudophakes.
- Dilate pupil maximally. Use minimum treatment – low power, least number of shots.
- Target areas of synechiae (peaked pupil) at pupillary edge. **Releasing adhesions will restore pupillary shape (sign of successful treatment). Intensive steroids are required to clear the inflammatory debris.**

10–35 shots (least necessary) × 1.0–1.5 mJ power (least necessary) × single shot × 0 defocus × Abraham's lens to synechiae or along the pupil margin.
- Treat with intensive steroids tapered over 6–8 weeks.

- Post-treatment steroids, mydriatics, and cycloplegics stabilize the blood-ocular barrier and prevent recurrences.
- Do not treat phakic patients with PS or inflammatory pupillary membranes as there is a risk of anterior capsular damage and phacolytic glaucoma from a leaky lens.

2.5.1 Clearance of Inflammatory IOL Deposits

- IOL deposits are common with recurrent uveitis, composed of giant cells, fibroblasts, and macrophages. They require treatment in severe cases, if involving the central visual axis, and affecting vision.

- Low power – 0.6–0.8 mJ × 20–30 shots to deposits × single shot × 0 defocus × Abraham's lens. Target larger IOL deposits directly to see it disperse.

- Intensive steroids drops are needed for a longer period (3–4 weeks) after treatment. The IOL deposits can recur with recurrent uveitis.

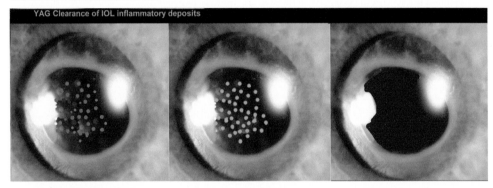

Figure 2.35 YAG clearance of inflammatory IOL deposits.

2.5.2 Clearance of Retained SLM in the Visual Axis

Retained cortical lens matter can occur after a difficult cataract surgery, associated with small pupils, small capsulorhexis, and PCR. It causes prolonged inflammation, corneal oedema, IOP elevation, and CMO, and promotes development of PCO.

Retained cortical lens matter identified in the immediate perioperative period should be removed surgically. Retained lens fragments with a PCR are best managed under the care of a VR surgeon.

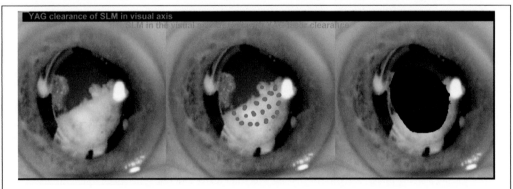

Figure 2.36 YAG clearance of SLM – 1.

SLM identified later requires treatment only if it affects the visual axis with symptoms.

Asymptomatic SLM sequestered peripherally in the capsular bag does not need treatment. A YAG posterior capsulotomy may dislodge SLM sequestered peripherally, causing it to drop into the visual axis.

YAG clearance is only required for the portion involving the central visual axis.
Surgical removal is indicated for large free-floating fragments in the AC, as they are unlikely to be amenable to YAG treatment and pose a risk for complications.

Laser treatment releases lens protein, causing inflammation and a rise in IOP, requiring **intensive treatment with anti-inflammatory drops, prophylactic anti-glaucoma therapy, and close monitoring after treatment.**

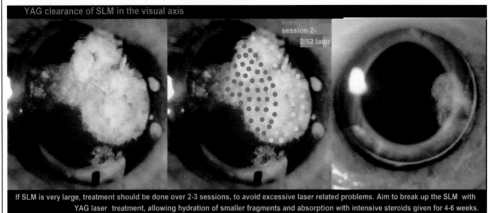

YAG clearance of SLM in the visual axis

session 2-
2/52 later

If SLM is very large, treatment should be done over 2-3 sessions, to avoid excessive laser related problems. Aim to break up the SLM with YAG laser treatment, allowing hydration of smaller fragments and absorption with intensive steroids given for 4-6 weeks.

Figure 2.37 YAG clearance of SLM – 2.

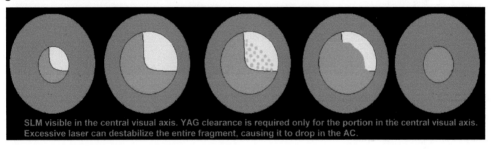

SLM visible in the central visual axis. YAG clearance is required only for the portion in the central visual axis. Excessive laser can destabilize the entire fragment, causing it to drop in the AC.

Figure 2.38 YAG clearance of SLM – diagrammatic.

Procedure is similar to YAG capsulotomy, with **higher power**.
Only treat the central visual axis. You do not need to treat the entire fragment.
20–30 shots × 2–4 mJ power × single shot × 0 defocus × Abraham's lens
Aim to break up SLM, allowing hydration of fragments in the AC and absorption with intensive steroids.
A larger fragment may need treatment over 2–3 sessions.

- **Excessive laser treatment can destabilize the entire fragment and cause a free- floating lens fragment in the AC, requiring surgical intervention.**

SUGGESTED READING

1. Karahan, E. et al. An overview of Nd:YAG laser capsulotomy, *Med Hypothesis Discov Innov Ophthalmol.* 2014;3(2):45–50.

2. Bhargava, R. et al. Nd-YAG laser capsulotomy energy levels for PCO. *J Ophthalmic Vis Res.* 2015;10(1):37–42.

3. Steinert, R. F. *Nd:YAG Laser Posterior Capsulotomy AAO* 4 Nov 2013.

4. Werner, L. et al. Causes of IOL opacification or discolouration. *J Cataract Refract Surg.* 2007;33:713–726.

5. Kim, J.S. et al. Comparison of two Nd-YAG laser posterior capsulotomy: cruciate pattern vs circular pattern with vitreous strand cutting. *Int J Ophthalmol.* 1984;10:182–184. doi: 10.18240/ijo.2018.02.09

6. Foot, L. et al. Surface calcification of Silicone plate IOL in patients with asteroid hyalosis. *Am J Ophthalmol.* 2004;137:979–987.

7. Ronbeck, M. et al. Comparison of PCO development with 3 IOL types: five-year prospective study. *J Cataract Refract Surg.* 2009;35(11):1935–1940. 10.1016/j.jcrs.2009.05.048.

8. Eliaçık, M. et al. Anterior segment OCT measurement after Nd-YAG laser capsulotomy. *Am J Ophthalmol.* 2014;158(5):994–998, 12 Aug 2014 PMID: 25127700.

9. Kim, H.K. et al. Capsular block syndrome after cataract surgery: clinical analysis and classification. *J Cataract Refract Surg.* 2008;34:357–363.

2.6 YAG LASER VITREOLYSIS

Nd-YAG laser is used to release vitreous strands to the corneal wounds following a complicated cataract surgery. This treatment is desirable due to the risk of persistent CMO and visual loss from **vitreous wick syndrome**.

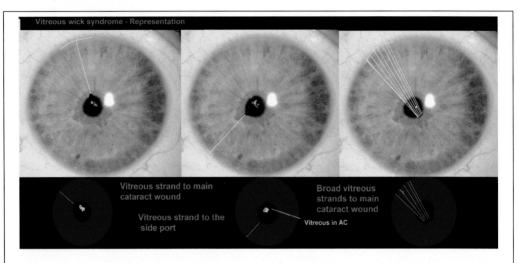

Figure 2.39 Vitreous wick syndrome.

Presentation of Vitreous Wick Syndrome
- History of complicated cataract surgery with PC rupture or zonular dehiscence.
- May have IOL mispositioning, vitreous in AC, peaked pupil, corneal oedema, chronic AC inflammation, and high IOP.
- Vitreous strand to main cataract wound or side port seen on clinical examination.
- Strands can be single and discrete, or multiple and broad, and may have iris adhesions or entrapment.
- Most patients have a low-grade ongoing post-operative uveitis.

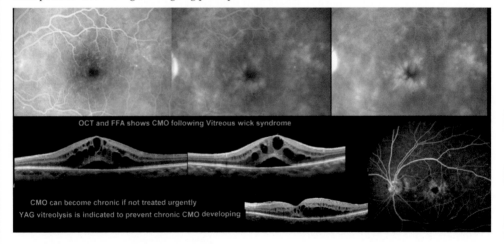

Figure 2.40 CMO with vitreous wick syndrome.

2.6.1 Treatment

The first line of treatment is preventative. Complicated cataract surgery, with vitreous loss, should have anterior vitrectomy to ensure vitreous wick does not develop, **confirmed by instilling pilocarpine drops to rule out a peaked pupil at the end of surgery.**

If vitreous wick is identified, **early treatment** (surgical or laser) is important to avoid development of CMO. Laser is considered less invasive and the preferred option.

Active post-operative inflammation must be treated prior to laser vitreolysis. Care must be taken in high myopes and patients with lattice degeneration, due to potential risk of retinal tears and detachment. Pre-existing CMO needs treatment with sub-tenon or peribulbar steroids.

2.6.2 YAG Vitreolysis for Vitreous Wick

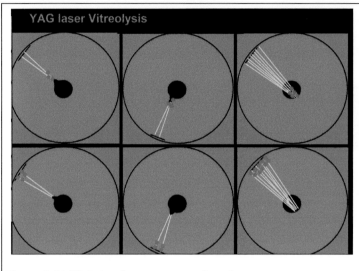

- Vitreous strand is targeted, either at the pupil margin or cataract wound, with good success.
- The narrowest point of vitreous attachment (easier to treat with minimum shots) and visibility of the vitreous wick dictates which site is appropriate.

Figure 2.41 YAG vitreolysis at cornea and pupil.

Vitreolysis at Cataract Wound

A cataract wound is a reliable landmark, easily visualized with an iridotomy or gonioscopy lens. Risks of vitreolysis in this area include corneal burns and endothelial injury with localized oedema (AC is narrower at the wound), and peripheral anterior synechiae, with excessive laser treatment.

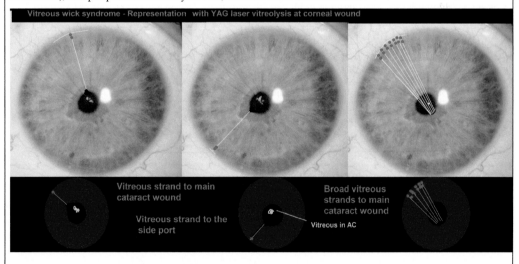

Figure 2.42 Vitreous wick syndrome with YAG vitreolysis at corneal wound.

Vitreolysis at the pupillary margin – easier to treat at the tip of peaked pupil.

The pupillary margin is a reliable landmark and safer area for treatment, as the AC is deep. A peaked pupil with a narrow band is easy to target. A broader band will need more shots. There is a small risk of iris injury and hyphema with poor focus.

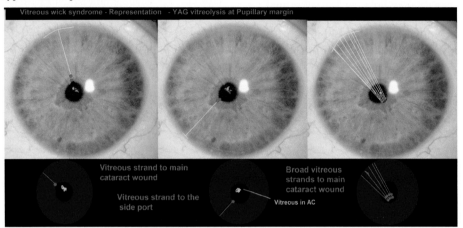

Figure 2.43 Vitreous wick syndrome with YAG vitreolysis at the pupillary margin.

Vitreolysis in the AC (Midway between 2 Ends)
- Usually not done, except if the vitreous strand has fibrosed and is clearly visible to focus on, with a deep AC. High risk of iris trauma, hyphema, and traumatic uveitis.

Vitreolysis Technique

- Informed consent is taken with risks/benefits explained.
- **Aim is to relieve vitreous traction, prevent CMO, stabilize vision, and restore pupil shape.**
- Patients are advised of risk of floaters, retinal detachment, persistent uveitis, CMO, secondary glaucoma, corneal oedema/scarring, and PAS.

Pre-laser Treatment
- **Pilocarpine 2% drops are used to constrict the pupil and stretch the vitreous strand to improve visibility and make treatment easy.**
- Topical apraclonidine reduces risk of an IOP spike.
- Select an **iridotomy lens with coupling fluid**. Use the magnifying button to focus on area of treatment.

Treatment
- **Switch on machine, set slit lamp parameters. Select YAG option.**
- **High magnification – ×16.**
- **Zero defocus.**
- **Single pulse.**
- **Higher power – 2–4 mJ** (vitreous is clear, with no pigment to absorb the laser energy).
- Aim just in front of the peaked pupil or the corneal wound.

- **Focus on the peaked pupil (iris) and then pull slit lamp slightly back to focus on the vitreous strand in the AC, without damaging the iris.**
- Number of shots will depend on width of the vitreous band. Generally, three to four shots for a single strand is adequate.
- With multiple bands, start treatment from the anterior-most band (in AC), and gradually move towards the iris.

Number of shots (based on width of band) × 2–4 mJ power × single pulse × 0 defocus × iridotomy lens. Start with lower power and gradually increase until reaction seen.
Treatment is successful if you note restoration of a round pupil.

Post Laser Treatment
- Apraclonidine prevents an IOP spike.
- Treatment may cause iris trauma with pigment release, inflammation, and hyphema, requiring treatment with mydriatics and anti-inflammatory (steroid) drops.
- Assessment of IOP after laser is essential, especially with difficult and prolonged treatment.
- Review patient in 2–3 weeks for an IOP assessment, fundal check, and OCT scan, to rule out CMO and RD.

SUGGESTED READING

1. Katzen, L.E. et al. YAG laser treatment of CMO. *Am J Ophthalmol*. 1983; May;95(5):589–592.

2. Steinert, R.F. et al. Nd:YAG laser anterior vitreolysis for Irvine-Gass CME. *J Cataract Refract Surg*. 1989;15(3):304–307.

3. Fankhauser, F. et al. Laser vitreolysis: a review. *Ophthalmologica*. 2002;Mar–Apr;216(2):73–84.

2.7 YAG LASER HYALOIDOTOMY

Blood trapped between ILM and posterior hyaloid face near the macula can cause severe visual loss. Spontaneous resolution can occur, but recovery is slow, causing prolonged visual disability, with risk of macular scarring.

A YAG laser can be used to clear a large, persistent, pre-macular subhyaloid bleed of more than three disc diameters.

Causes of Subhyaloid Haemorrhage
- Retinal vascular disorders such as PDR, RVO, RAM, ARMD, AV shunts
- Haematological disorders – aplastic anaemia, leukaemia
- Valsalva retinopathy, Terson's syndrome, Purtscher's retinopathy, trauma

Treatment of Subhyaloid Haemorrhage
- A small haemorrhage is treated conservatively and usually resolves spontaneously.
- A large haemorrhage requires treatment to release the sequestered pre-macular blood and reduce risk of macular scarring and ERM.
- Puncturing the posterior hyaloid face with a Q-switch Nd:YAG laser releases trapped blood into the vitreous cavity, facilitating absorption.
- **PRP, for underlying vascular aetiology, should be completed prior to YAG laser hyaloidotomy.** This is important as hyaloidotomy will induce a vitreous haemorrhage, preventing a clear fundal view for PRP.

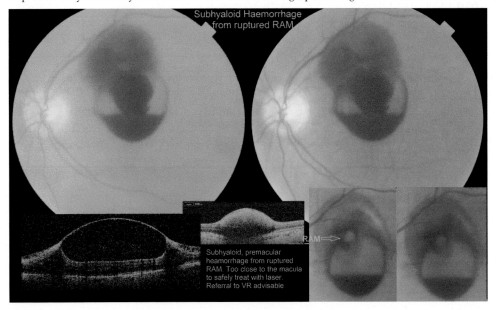

Figure 2.44 Subhyaloid haemorrhage.

Vitreoretinal referral for vitrectomy is required for:
- Persistent vitreous haemorrhage.
- Failure of YAG hyaloidotomy (persistent sub-macular haemorrhage).
- Pre-retinal fibrosis (epiretinal membrane), macular pucker and visual distortion.

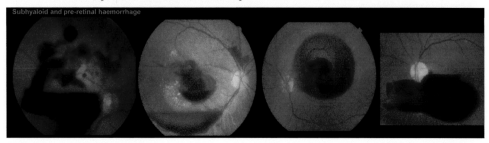

Subhyaloid and pre-retinal haemorrhage

Figure 2.45 Subhyaloid and preretinal haemorrhage.

2.7.1 Procedure

Consent must be detailed and clear. The aim is to release trapped blood. Visual improvement is not guaranteed, and visual prognosis is guarded, especially in long-standing cases. Laser will induce a vitreous haemorrhage, worsening vision loss initially, and if persistent may require further treatment with VR surgery.

2.7.1.1 Pre-treatment Drops

- Dilate both eyes (tropicamide 1% and phenylephrine 2.5%).
- Apraclonidine is used to prevent an IOP spike, and a **Mainster Focal or Area Centralis lens** is used with a coupling agent and topical anaesthetic.

2.7.1.2 Treatment

- Identify the inferior demarcation of the subhyaloid haemorrhage.
- **Create an opening in the posterior hyaloid membrane just above the inferior margin of the haemorrhage** (to have a cushion of blood, to protect underlying retina), **away from the fovea or retinal blood vessels.**
- **Start with 3 mJ power, and gradually increase by 1mJ until a perforation is visible at the surface and blood drains under gravity into the vitreous cavity (power range is 3–11 mJ).**

3–8 shots × 5–8 mJ power × single pulse × 0 defocus × Mainster Focal lens. Abandon after 5–8 shots if unsuccessful. Refer to VR surgery.

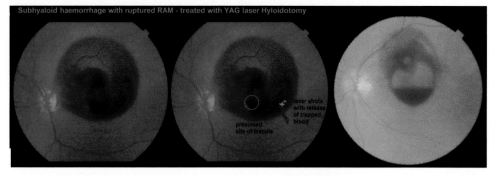

Subhyaloid haemorrhage with ruptured RAM - treated with YAG laser Hyloidotomy

presumed site of macula

laser shots with release of trapped blood

Figure 2.46 Subhyaloid haemorrhage treated with YAG hyaloidotomy.

SUGGESTED READING

1. Menne, S. Subhyaloidal and macular haemorrhage: localisation and treatment strategies. *Br J Ophthalmol.* 2007 Jul; 91(7):850–852. doi: 10.1136/bjo.2007.114025

2. Raymond, L.A. Nd-YAG laser treatment for haemorrhages under the ILM and posterior hyaloid face in macula. *Ophthalmology.* 1995;Mar;102(3):406–411. doi: 10.1016/s0161-6420(95)31008-1.PMID: 7891977 Clinical Trial.

Section 3 Lasers in Glaucoma

This section looks at laser treatments in glaucoma including the three common procedures, laser iridotomy, iridoplasty, and SLT. It aims to clarify understanding, improve laser techniques, and handle complications associated with these treatments.

3.1 INTRODUCTION

Glaucoma is a chronic progressive condition, causing pressure-related optic neuropathy. Treatment can be broadly categorized as:

- Medical management (topical and oral agents) – this can be associated with compliance issues, local or systemic side effects, and adverse surgical outcomes.
- Laser treatment.

- Surgical treatments that are more invasive and expensive.

Lasers in glaucoma are used for diagnostic (OCT, SLO, HRT) and therapeutic purposes. Therapeutic lasers are broadly divided into:

3.1.1 Outflow Enhancing Procedures

- Trabeculoplasty.
- Peripheral iridotomy.
- Iridoplasty.

3.1.2 Inflow Reducing Procedures (Aqueous Production)

- Cyclophotocoagulation and other less common laser procedures.

Presentation	Common laser procedures for IOP control
Narrow occludable angles ACG (primary/secondary) Plateau iris syndrome	LPI to prevent pupil block LPI to relieve pupil block LPI to alter iris contour
Postoperative laser	Post-trabeculectomy suture lysis Sclerostomy if not patent Gonio-puncture if not patent
OHT, early POAG	SLT – 1st line (avoid topical therapy)
POAG with poor response or side-effects to topical treatment	SLT – 2nd line (adjunct to drops or surgery)
Malignant glaucoma	Capsulotomy and disruption of anterior hyaloid face in pseudophakic patient
End-stage glaucoma, NVG	Cyclophotocoagulation – reduce aqueous formation (external – cyclodiode, or internal – endo-cyclophotocoagulation)

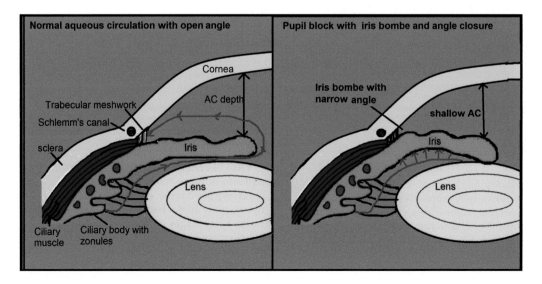

Figure 3.1 Diagram of ocular angle

DOI: 10.1201/9781003144304-4

3.2 YAG LASER PERIPHERAL IRIDOTOMY (LPI)

Narrow angles refer to irido-trabecular apposition, due to **pupil block or lens induced factors**. Presentation varies from asymptomatic narrowing (narrow angles with no symptoms) to a full-blown attack of angle closure.

The incidence is around 1% of the general population but is higher in Inuit Eskimo and Asians (thick iris). Increasing age, female gender, hypermetropia, and developing cataracts are added risk factors.

Not every narrow angle is occludable, and detailed examination, including gonioscopy, is essential to identify those at risk.

YAG LPI creates an alternative route for aqueous flow and opens the angle.

Van Herrick Classification of Angle			
Grade	Degree	Risk of AACG	Description
0	0	AACG attack	Closed angle
1	10	High risk of ACG	Highly occludable angle
2	20	Moderate risk of ACG	Likely occludable angle
3	21-35	Unlikely to get ACG	Reasonably open angle
4	>35	No risk of ACG	Widely open angle
Grade 0 is acute attack; Grades 1 and 2 are angles at risk of closure and need LPI.			

3.2.1 Indications for YAG LPI

Prophylactic LPI   • **Narrow occludable angles in 2 or more quadrants.**   • **History of intermittent subacute attacks of ACG or ACG in other eye.**
Therapeutic LPI   • **Treat attack of primary AACG.**   • **Chronic ACG** – prognosis is worse due to presence of PAS and optic neuropathy.   • **Plateau iris syndrome with steep iris insertion and narrow angles.**
Secondary Pupil Block (Secondary ACG)   *LPI relieves pupil block, allowing a safer lensectomy.*   • **Secondary pupil block** – iris cyst, occlusio pupillae due to PS (*posterior synechiae*), incomplete surgical PI, inflammatory pupillary membrane, nanophthalmos, silicone oil after vitrectomy.   • Malignant glaucoma (aqueous misdirection).   • **Lens related** – cataract – senile or traumatic (phacomormic), dislocated or subluxated lens (ectopia lentis), pseudophakia with dislocated IOL, pupil block with ACIOL (if PI absent or blocked),   • **Non-pupil block ACG** – uveitis with PAS, cyclitic membrane, iris incarceration, epithelial ingrowth, retrolental fibrous membrane, RD, choroidal effusion, VKH.   • **To alter iris configuration in PDS and break reverse pupil block.**

When Should LPI Not Be Done?	
Absolute contraindications	**Relative contraindications**
• Extensive corneal oedema or opacity – AC and iris not visible. • Flat anterior chamber. • Conditions causing extensive synechial angle closure including neovascular glaucoma and iridocorneal endothelial (ICE) syndrome.	• Limited view – corneal oedema, opacity, aqueous haze. • Chronic uveitis. • Early NVI. • Bleeding disorders, anti-coagulants. • Nystagmus. • Poor co-operation mobility, difficult positioning, blepharospasm.

3.2.2 How Does YAG LPI Work?

Primary ACG increases IOP by impaired outflow due to appositional (acute phase) or synechial (chronic phase) closure of the AC angle. The underlying mechanism is **primary pupillary block**, which stops aqueous flow, builds pressure in the posterior chamber, causing iris bombe, complete angle closure, and precipitating an acute attack. In secondary ACG, the pupil block is secondary to other underlying causes.

YAG PI creates an alternative route for aqueous outflow, relieving pupil block, reversing iris bombe, deepening the AC, and opening the angle. **Iridotomy is most effective in the early stages of the disease**. It is less effective once extensive synechiae and optic neuropathy have developed.

Laser peripheral iridotomy (LPI) is performed with the **Q-switched Nd-YAG laser (1064nm wavelength), using the principle of photo-disruption.** The Q-switch enables

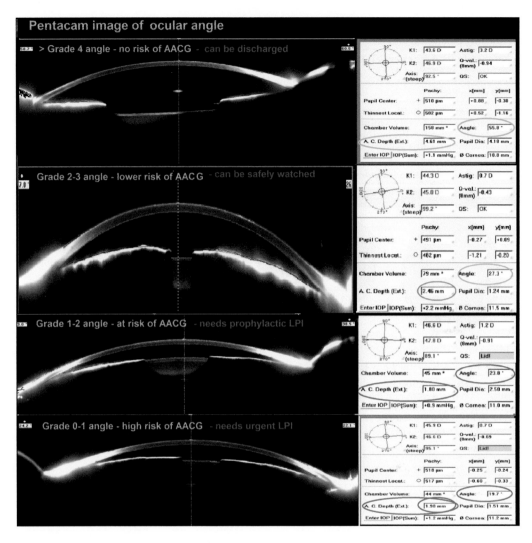

Figure 3.2 Pentacam images of ocular angle.

production of an extremely short, high-powered laser pulse, ideal for photo-disruption, with no thermal effect, and low failure, or complication rates than photothermal lasers. YAG iridotomies are less likely to close over time and work better with lighter, thinner irises. The laser ionizes tissue creating a rapidly expanding plasma and cavitation bubble with an explosive effect, leading to shockwaves that cause tissue disruption.

3.2.3 Laser Peripheral Iridotomy – Procedure

> **Patient examination prior to procedure, includes:**
> - BCVA (*best corrected VA*), IOP (*intraocular pressure*), corneal assessment.
> - AC depth, gonioscopy to assess the grade and pigmentation of angle.
> - Iris configuration and vasculature.
> - presence of PAS, pigment dispersion.
> - Causes of secondary pupil block.
> - Co-existing ocular problems that may affect procedure or prognosis – cataract, uveitis, zonular weakness, iridodonesis, vitreoretinal pathology.
> - **Systemic problems** – bleeding disorders, patients on anticoagulants, head tremors.
>
> **Avoid LPI with extremely high IOP – increased risk of complications.**
> - High IOP causes corneal oedema and iris congestion, making the procedure difficult with high risk of bleeding, hyphema, and treatment failure. High IOP should be treated with medical therapy prior to laser.

Anticipation and preparation are key. It is important to seek help when necessary (anxious patients, positioning problems).

- **Informed consent is essential. The aim of treatment is to reverse pupil block, open the angle, and abate or prevent an attack of ACG.**
- Patients must be warned of risk of treatment failure, bleeding, high IOP, inflammation, repeat treatments, and vision loss.

Pre-treatment with miotics – improves efficacy and safety profile of treatment.
- **Pilocarpine 2% ×3, every 5 minutes, to the eye for treatment.**
- **Pilocarpine stretches the peripheral iris, making it thin and easier to perforate.**
- **Apraclonidine (alpha-agonist) or other topical glaucoma drops are used to prevent an IOP spike.** Ensure pre-laser IOP is stable.

Lens selection – Abraham iridotomy lens used with topical anaesthetic and coupling lubricant.

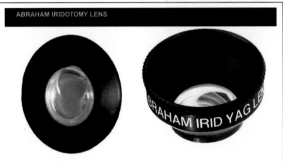

ABRAHAM IRIDOTOMY LENS

Abraham Lens
Convex button enlarges laser spot at the cornea, reducing risk of corneal burns (collateral damage), and focuses (reduces spot) on the iris. This reduces the energy requirement, increasing power density, improving laser effect, and making treatment safer. The power density at the iris is four times greater than at the cornea.

Figure 3.3 Abraham iridotomy lens.

Slit lamp settings – adjust the:
- IPD and refractive error on the slit lamp eye-piece, and the table height.
- **Use lower magnification to view and higher magnification (×16) for treatment.**
- Use full slit height, moderate slit width, and just visible slit lamp and aiming beam brightness.
- **Switch on laser, and select YAG from home page.**

Setting the Laser Parameters

- **Defocus – set at zero.** This means you deliver laser energy at the point of focus.

- **Power – set at 1.5–3 mJ depending on thickness of the iris.**

- **Pulse – select triple shots (total Power – 1.5 – 3 mJ × 3 = 4.5 mJ – 9 mJ).**

If single shot selected, start with higher power, and more shots will be needed.

Focus on anterior iris stroma (just behind the iris surface).

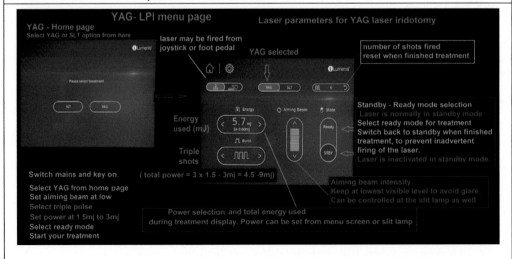

Figure 3.4 YAG LPI menu page.

- **Site selection is vital to ensure a successful PI.**
- A site between 11 and 1 o'clock is preferred as PI holes are covered by the upper lid and patients do not experience diplopia or glare from polycoria.
- **Choose a small iris crypt or thin iris area, as peripheral as possible.**

Why is it essential to select a peripheral site?

A miosed pupil (with pilocarpine) causes iris stretch, which is maximum in the periphery. **The iris is thinnest and easiest to perforate in the periphery**.

To achieve maximum miosis and iris stretch, pilocarpine 2% is instilled three times at 5–10-minute intervals prior to treatment.

A mid-peripheral site is best avoided – this involves going through the belly of the muscle, which is thicker, requiring higher energy, more shots, with a higher risk of iris bleed and hitting the lens capsule behind. In addition, an LPI in the mid-periphery is liable to become occluded during pupillary dilatation. **Large crypts are usually associated with blood vessels at their edges and are best avoided**.

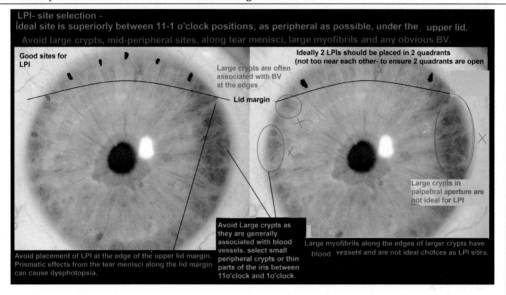

Figure 3.5 LPI site selection.

Number of Iridotomies

- **A single well-done LPI in an appropriate location is generally accepted as adequate treatment, especially for prophylaxis.**
- **Some** (*author included*) **advocate making 2 LPI holes at 11 o'clock and 1 o'clock positions, especially in CACG with PAS and plateau iris.** A single PI may not completely open the angle and still poses a significant risk of AACG. **Doing 2 PIs ensures that at least 2 quadrants of the angle are open, reducing risk of an acute attack.**

Treatment Procedure

- Focus on a peripheral iris crypt or thin iris area, anywhere between the 11 and 1 o'clock position, avoiding any obvious blood vessels (often at the edge of large crypts).
- **Select ready mode** – YAG laser will show 2 red lights – **aiming beam.**
- Align the 2 aiming beams to a single spot just behind the iris surface.
- You are now ready to fire your shot.
- 3–4 (×3) shots are generally adequate to complete a single PI.
- **A small (150–200 μm) full-thickness peripheral hole is the ideal endpoint**.
- **A gush of pigment and fluid from the posterior chamber or lens visualization through the iridotomy suggests permeability.**
- A patent PI transilluminates, but this may be difficult to assess with media opacities.

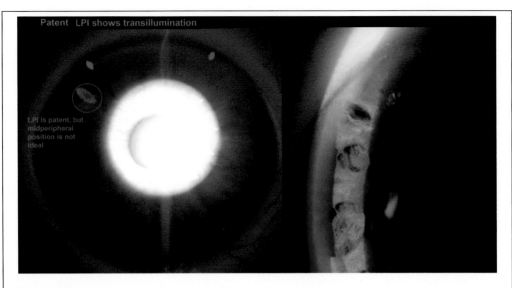

Figure 3.6 Patent LPI.

Laser Parameters for LPI
3–4 (x3) shots × 1.5–3 mJ power × triple pulse × 0 defocus × Abraham lens
Power selected is 1.5–3 mJ ×3 = total of 4.5–9 mJ for each PI.
Thin iris – 4.5 mJ is adequate. Thick iris or no peripheral crypt – needs higher power.
Avoid any obvious surface blood vessels, usually at the edge of large crypts.

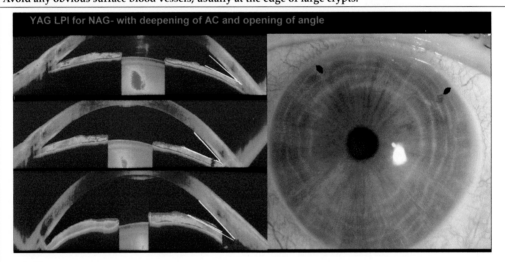

Figure 3.7 YAG LPI -1.

Post-Treatment
Apraclonidine (Iopidine) prevents an IOP spike. LPI patency and IOP are reviewed in an hour. Patients are discharged on steroid drops over the next 1–2 weeks. Intensive treatment is required with excessive inflammation or a hyphema.
- Primary AACG – pre-existing glaucoma drops can be stopped after LPI, provided it is patent.
- If patency cannot be assured, it is safer to continue the drops, until review. Patients are asked to stop drops 1–2 days prior to their assessment.
- CACG with optic neuropathy need to continue with their glaucoma drops long term.
- Follow up is arranged in 2–4 weeks, to confirm successful treatment.

3.2.4 Complications of LPI

Iris Haemorrhage/Hyphema (30–50% – common after LPI)
- Due to poor site selection (mid-periphery, large crypts) and use of high energy.
- Higher risk with engorged blood vessels, associated with AACG, persistent high IOP, uveitis, bleeding disorders, and patients on anticoagulants.
- **YAG does not cauterize blood vessels as photothermal lasers.**
- May cause IOP elevation, inflammation, and reduced vision if involving the visual axis.

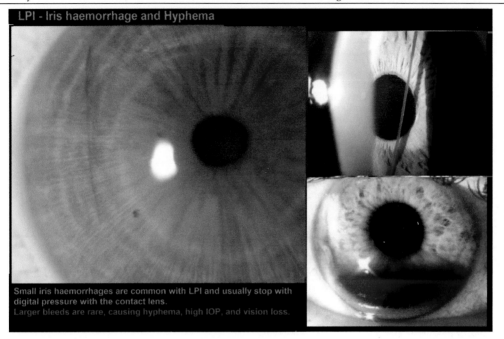

LPI - Iris haemorrhage and Hyphema

Small iris haemorrhages are common with LPI and usually stop with digital pressure with the contact lens.
Larger bleeds are rare, causing hyphema, high IOP, and vision loss.

Figure 3.8 LPI with iris haemorrhage and hyphema.

Treatment
- Site selection is vital. Avoid obvious surface blood vessels or large crypts.
- **If a bleed occurs, stop treatment, and press firmly with the contact lens.** Most bleeds stop with digital pressure from the lens.
- **Re-site the LPI once the bleed has stopped. Do not treat the same area again.**
- Rarely, with persistent bleed causing a hyphema, the procedure may need to be abandoned. LPI can be completed once the hyphema has cleared, with appropriate medical treatment.
- **Bleeding can be limited by pre-treating the proposed site with a photothermal laser (argon/PASCAL). This is useful in patients with known coagulative disorder or on anticoagulants.**

Corneal injury/burns
Isolated corneal burns cause temporary cloudy swelling (ground glass appearance), which usually clears spontaneously, with no long-term effects.
- Poor focus results in localized stromal injury and focal corneal opacity.
- Endothelial damage with reduced endothelial cell count can occur after LPI (common with argon laser) causing persistent corneal oedema.

More likely with:
- **Very shallow AC, extremely narrow angles, plateau iris, and corneal oedema.**
- **Use of excessive power, not using a contact lens, poor focus, poor site selection, and excessive patient movement.**

Treatment
- Reduce power used – **always use a contact lens.** Select a crypt or thin part of iris, as peripheral as possible (requires less energy). Focus slightly behind the iris surface (in anterior stroma – lower risk of burns).
- **Do not treat the same area again – risk of inducing PAS.**
- **Re-site PI if corneal clouding obscures your view.**

Inflammation
- Post-laser inflammation is common and usually settles with a topical steroid.
- Worse with higher energy, excessive shots, midperipheral PI (thicker muscle), and pre-existing inflammatory eye diseases.

Treatment
- Appropriate site selection, conservative treatment, and use intensive steroids for longer periods with excessive or pre-existing inflammation.

IOP elevation
Transient IOP spike is common after LPI, usually mild, short-lasting (<24 hours), due to release of pigment, blood, and debris clogging up TM or incomplete iridotomy.
Persistent IOP elevation is more common in:
- Asian/African eyes.
- Use of higher energy, more shots per treatment.
- With advanced CACG – extensive synechial closure of angle.
- Mixed mechanism or secondary pupil block glaucoma.
- Unrecognized plateau iris syndrome.
- Other non-pupillary block glaucoma, secondary to inflammation, hyphema, and prolonged corticosteroid therapy.

Treatment
- Apraclonidine (Iopidine), pre- and post-treatment, prevents an IOP spike.
- Persistent rise may need anti-glaucoma treatment.
- **If angle remains narrow – consider plateau iris, needing iridoplasty or long-term pilocarpine drops.**
- Treatment of associated uveitis, hyphema, other causes of secondary pupil block.
- Consider lensectomy if cataract or swollen lens is causing pupil block.
- LPI can overwhelm an already compromised TM, causing sustained and severe IOP elevation, precipitating need for filtration surgery (trabeculectomy, stents, tubes).

Lens capsule damage, cataract acceleration, and zonular damage

- Associated with mid-peripheral site, poor focus, not using CL, using power >10mJ, poor patient co-operation positioning, and excessive movement.
- **Treating via a patent or partially patent PI in a redo PI (when treating a partially patent PI or enlarging a patent PI) carries a higher risk of lens capsule damage, cataract acceleration, and zonular damage.**
- **Accelerated cataract formation** – due to direct damage to lens capsule causes iritis, altered aqueous dynamics, metabolic lens changes.
- **Risk of phacolytic glaucoma, from a leaking lens.**
- Patients with pre-existing zonular weakness or dehiscence, or a subluxated or dislocated lens have a higher risk of lenticular or zonular damage.

Treatment
- Focus is critical. Always use a contact lens (fixates eye, magnifies view, reduces power needed). Ensure good head position and eye fixation.
- **Do not apply laser via the pupil or a patent PI.**
- **If retreating a partially patent PI use lower power and single shots.**
- **Iridotomy should always be placed in the periphery, beyond the anterior lens curvature (distance between the iris and anterior lens capsule is greatest).**

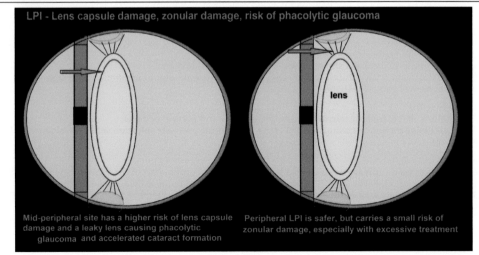

Figure 3.9 LPI lens capsule damage.

Dysphotopsia (6–12%)
- Visual symptoms of glare, haloes, ghost images are rare, and more likely with partially or fully exposed iridotomies, large PI, or PI along the upper tear menisci (prismatic effect).

Treatment – site selection is vital
- Ensure PI are not too large, extremely peripheral, and fully covered by upper lids.
- Some users suggest placing PI in the palpebral aperture (at 3 and 9 o'clock position). This has no proven benefit, but an increased risk of polycoria related problems.

Incomplete PI/closure of PI
- Commonly due to failure to perforate, and rarely due to late closure. Mid-peripheral PI are more likely to close, especially on dilation.
- More common with thick, dark iris (difficult to penetrate, higher risk of bleeding).

Treatment
- Some patients may require a second attempt within a few days (**absolute failure is unusual with YAG lasers**). If patency is doubtful, treatment options include choosing a new site or enlarging the initial opening.
- Enlarging iridotomies, although potentially hazardous, can be accomplished by lower power, fewer shots, single pulses.

Other rare complications
- Retinal burns, cystoid macular oedema, malignant glaucoma, floaters, loss of vision, retinal tears, and detachment especially in nanophthalmic eyes.
- **CL-related problem.**

Argon / PASCAL Laser Iridoplasty + Iridotomy – rarely done due to higher complication risks (corneal burns, PAS, inflammation, retinal injury, higher closure, and failure rates).

3.2.5 Sequential Argon/PASCAL Iridoplasty with Nd:YAG PI

Penetrating a thick, dark iris can be difficult, requiring high power, with a greater risk of complications. Photothermal iridoplasty can be used to pre-treat and thin the iris stroma at the LPI site, making YAG PI easier.

Additionally, photothermal lasers coagulate iris vessels, reducing the risk of hyphema. This is advantageous in patients with engorged vessels or bleeding disorders, or on anticoagulants.

Preparation same as for LPI.	
Argon or PASCAL laser Iridoplasty **Power – 200–500 mw – see iris contract.** **Spot size – 200 μm** **Pulse duration – 20–40 ms (long)** Apply 4–6 shots to peripheral LPI site using an iridotomy lens.	**Nd-YAG laser Peripheral Iridotomy** **Power – 1.5–3 mJ × 3 (triple burst) = total power of 4.5–9 mJ.** **Defocus – zero** Apply YAG to the area of iridoplasty, using an iridotomy lens.

3.2.6 Outcomes of LPI

PI successful – no additional treatment required. • **Anatomical improvement** – deepening of AC, opening of angles. • Iridotomy relieves attack in 65–72% of Caucasians with AACG. • Review in 2 weeks, 6 months, then discharge to opticians for yearly monitoring.

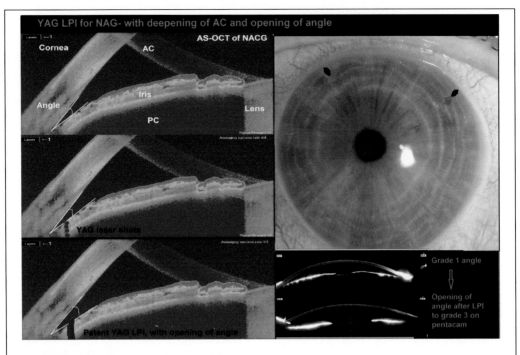

Figure 3.10 YAG LPI -2.

Failed PI – additional medical or surgical intervention needed.
- **PI is not patent and IOP remains high – repeat laser treatment**.
- **PI is patent but angle remains narrow**
  - Consider **plateau iris** – pilocarpine drops or laser iridoplasty required.

  IOP remains high – consider
  - **Additional glaucoma medication.**
  - **Lensectomy.**
  - **Filtration surgery.**
  - **Treatment for co-existent problems** – uveitis, steroid responder.

PI is more effective in early stages of PAC spectrum.
- **Higher IOP (>35 mmHg), longer attack duration, poor initial response (<30% IOP drop), extensive PAS (>6 clock hours), and established optic neuropathy affect outcomes adversely needing further medical or surgical interventions**.
- **Presence of PAS is a worse prognostic indicator, suggestive of chronicity.**
- **Asian and African patients have high IOP (>20% in 1 year and almost 60% in 4 years), with worse outcomes**. *(Due to anatomical variations in angle configuration, anterior lens position, plateau iris, need for higher power due to darker iris, severity, and duration of AAC attack and possible late presentation.)*

Close monitoring is therefore advised for all patients, even after a successful LPI.

- **Role of lensectomy in management of primary angle closure** – lens extraction is effective in deepening the AC and relieving pupil block. However, surgery carries a risk and should only be considered if LPI is not effective.
- **Patients with lens-related pupil block should have an LPI prior to cataract surgery (LPI makes lensectomy safer).**

- **Consider filtration surgery if all treatment fails.**

3.3 PIGMENT DISPERSION SYNDROME (PDS)

PDS is characterized by pigment loss from posterior iris surface, causing mid-peripheral iris transillumination defects, with pigment deposition on the lens surface, corneal endothelium, and trabecular meshwork (TM). PDS is commonly prevalent in white males in the third or fourth decade of life. It can be inherited and is more common in myopes.

PDS may be associated with normal or elevated IOP (due to pigment blocking TM), without optic neuropathy. Patients with optic nerve damage or visual field defect are classified as pigmentary glaucoma.

The **proposed mechanism of PDS is posterior bowing of iris (reverse pupillary block) causing irido-lenticular touch and iris**

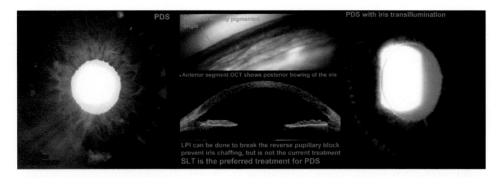

Figure 3.11 PDS.

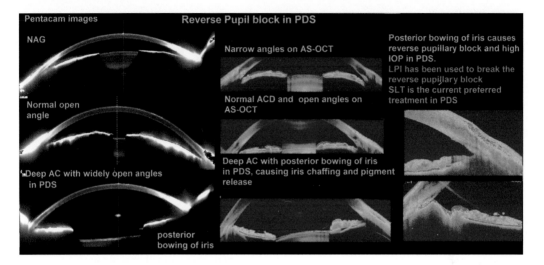

Figure 3.12 Reverse pupillary block in PDS.

chaffing, leading to pigment release. **Laser peripheral iridotomy has been used to break a reverse pupillary block.**

Studies have shown that LPI reverses the concave iris configuration, breaks reverse pupillary block, and reduces iris-lens chaffing, to reduce pigment release, but does not stop progression of pigmentary glaucoma. **LPI is not current standard practice in PDS.**

SLT offers better response for PDS glaucoma, due to pigmented angle. (*Discussed in section 3.5*).

3.4 PLATEAU IRIS

Plateau iris is a variant ACG, presenting in **younger hyperopic, female patients**, in their 30–50s, often with a family history of angle-closure glaucoma. Slit lamp examination shows normal central AC depth with a flat or slightly convex iris surface.

Gonioscopy reveals an extremely narrow angle, with steep anterior iris insertion.

Indentation gonioscopy shows the double-hump sign. The peripheral hump is due to the ciliary body propping up the iris root, and the central hump represents the central third of the iris resting over the anterior lens surface. More force is needed to open the angle on indentation gonioscopy than with pupillary block angle closure.

3.4.1 Mechanism of Glaucoma

- Presence of a large or anteriorly positioned ciliary body mechanically alters the position of the peripheral iris in relation to the trabecular meshwork.

- The iris root is inserted anteriorly on the ciliary face, further crowding the angle and obstructing aqueous flow via the TM, leading to angle-closure.

- Associated element of pupillary block.

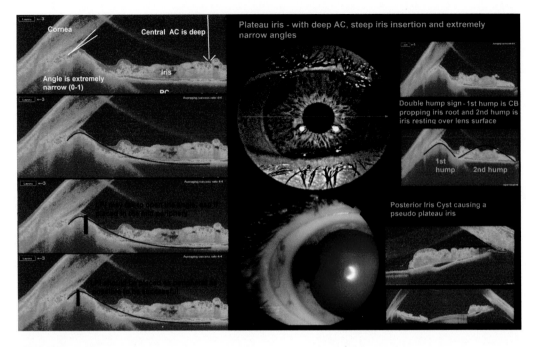

Figure 3.13 Plateau iris.

YAG laser iridotomy should always be performed as the first intervention.

Plateau iris should be suspected if angle remains narrow, despite a patent PI, and diagnosis is confirmed by gonioscopy and angle imaging with AS-OCT or UBM.

3.4.1.1 Treatment and Outcome

■ **Laser iridotomy should be performed as peripherally as possible.**

■ **Pilocarpine may produce iris thinning and facilitate angle opening.**

■ **LPI may not significantly alter angle anatomy**, and further treatment may be needed with:

■ Laser iridoplasty – to alter shape of peripheral iris and open the angle.

■ Long-term pilocarpine drops especially if IOP raised.

■ Periodic gonioscopy important (angle may narrow further with age).

3.5 IRIDOPLASTY

Iridoplasty is a technique used to reshape peripheral iris, break PAS, and pull the iris away from the trabecular meshwork, to open a crowded angle and improve outflow in patients with plateau iris syndrome, using low energy from a photothermal laser (Argon or PASCAL). It is also used to coagulate and thin a localized area of iris prior to an LPI in patients with thick irises or bleeding disorders.

Indications for Iridoplasty Treatment of Non-Pupil Block Glaucoma
• Plateau iris.
• Microphthalmos, nanophthalmos, presence of PAS – compromised angle, which worsens with developing cataract.
• Large iris and ciliary body cysts causing localized appositional angle closure.
• Iridoplasty in CACG is controversial but appears to reduce risk of PAS formation and help break early PAS (due to contraction of peripheral iris).

Localized iridoplasty – pre-treatment to LPI, in patients with dark brown iris, and coagulate blood vessels at the LPI site in patients with bleeding disorders, to reduce risk of hyphema.

It is easily performed, without requiring precise focus, with reasonable long-term outcomes. **It can be done in patients with corneal oedema where an LPI may be difficult**.

An initial iridoplasty may open the angle, reducing IOP and corneal oedema, to allow a safe LPI subsequently. It may prevent PAS formation, from prolonged appositional angle closure in an inflamed eye, and open a narrow angle to allow SLT treatment.

Mechanism of Action

A series of thermal burns placed in the peripheral iris (Argon or PASCAL), cause iris stroma to contract and pull away from angle structures, break PAS, and facilitate a **mechanical widening of the angle recess**. In plateau iris, heating and shrinkage thins, flattens, and reshapes the peripheral iris.

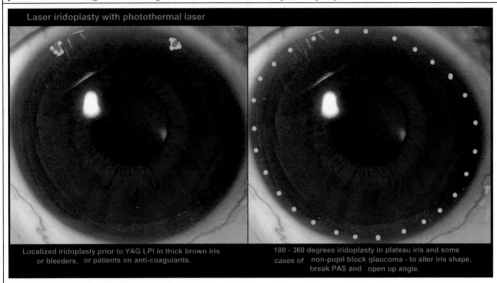

Laser iridoplasty with photothermal laser

Localized iridoplasty prior to YAG LPI in thick brown iris or bleeders, or patients on anti-coagulants.

180 - 360 degrees iridoplasty in plateau iris and some cases of non-pupil block glaucoma - to alter iris shape, break PAS and open up angle.

Figure 3.14 Laser iridoplasty.

Laser settings – PASCAL – single spot
Spot size – large – 200–400 μm
Pulse duration – long – 20–40 ms
Power – 200–500 mW (until you see iris tissue contract).
Treat 180–360 degrees, 5–8 burns/quadrant spaced evenly. Total of 20–30 shots with a gap of 2 spot sizes between burns, avoiding visible blood vessel.
If bubbles form or pigment is released, reduce the power.

Technique
Pre-treatment drops
• **Pilocarpine 2%, constricts pupil and stretches the iris**
• **Brimonidine or Iopidine to prevent IOP spike**
• **Topical anaesthetic with CL.**
Direct technique – using Abraham iridotomy lens to focus on peripheral iris.
Indirect technique – using gonio mirror to view the peripheral iris, angle, TM.

Iopidine prevents an IOP spike, and a course of topical steroids reduces inflammation. Periodic gonioscopy and IOP review is important, to rule out future angle narrowing.

Complications	Reasons for failure
• Low-grade inflammation.	• Inadequate treatment.
• IOP spike.	• Ineffective energy selection.
• Corneal endothelial burn.	• Improper site selection.
• Rarely, dilated, distorted pupil, iris haemorrhage or necrosis with heavy laser.	• Improper application.
• Failure of treatment/retreatment.	• Presence of PAS.

Do not perform iridoplasty for PAS resulting from uveitic glaucoma and neovascular glaucoma.

SUGGESTED READING

1. GLT Research Group. The Glaucoma Laser Trial (GLT) and GLT follow-up study: results. *Am J Ophthalmol.* 1995;120(6):718–731.

2. He, M. et al. LPI peripheral iridotomy in primary angle-closure suspects: biometric and gonioscopic outcomes: the Liwan Eye Study. *Ophthalmology.* 2007;114(3): 494–500.

3. Robin, A.L. et al. Argon laser PI in the treatment of PACG. *Arch Ophthalmol.* 1982;100: 919–923.

4. Ang, L.P. et al. Acute primary angle closure in an Asian population: long-term outcome of the fellow eye after prophylactic laser peripheral iridotomy. *Ophthalmology.* 2000;107:2092–2096.

5. Friedman, D.S. *Who needs an iridotomy?.* http://dx.doi.org/10.1136/bjo.85.9.1019

6. Bourdon, H. et al. Iridoplasty for plateau iris syndrome: a systematic review. *Open Ophthalmology*, 2019. http://dx.doi.org/10.1136/bmjophth-2019-000340

7. Tarongoy, P. et al. ACG: the role of the lens in the pathogenesis, prevention, and treatment. *Surv Ophthalmol.* 2009;54:211–225.

8. Nolan, W.P. et al. YAG LPI treatment for PACG in east Asian eyes. *Br J Ophthalmol.* 2000. Nov;84(11):1255–1259. doi: 10.1136/bjo.84.11.1255.

9. Lim, S.H. Clinical applications of anterior segment OCT. *J Ophthalmol.* 2015;2015:605729.

3.6 SELECTIVE LASER TRABECULOPLASTY (SLT)

Selective laser trabeculoplasty is a technique to stimulate aqueous drainage and improve IOP control in primary open angle glaucoma.

SLT works by selectively targeting intracellular pigment (melanin) within the trabecular meshwork cells, with a Q-switched, frequency doubled KTP-YAG photothermal laser, using 532nm (green visible) wavelength.

Thermal relaxation time (TRT) is the time taken for heat generated by photothermal laser to dissipate to surrounding tissues by 60% and dictates the extent of tissue damage. Long tissue exposure to laser energy (high TRT) is associated with more scarring and damage. This was the major limiting problem with argon laser trabeculoplasty (ALT). The Q-switch reduces pulse duration to less than TRT of melanin in the pigmented TM cells (2us).

SLT has a pulse duration of 3 nanoseconds, which is significantly less than TRT of TM cellular pigment, preventing transfer of heat to the surrounding tissues, sparing them from damage, making SLT an extremely safe, effective, and repeatable treatment in POAG.

3.6.1 SLT vs ALT

SLT is a safer procedure in comparison to ALT.			
	SLT	**ALT**	**Ratio**
Number of spots/ 180°	50	50	1:1
Spot size	400 μm (large) – diffuses energy	50 μm (small) – concentrates energy	8:1
Pulse duration	3 ns (v. short)	0.1 sec (long)	1:10^9
Energy	0.6–1.4 mJ (low)	400–600 mw (v. high)	1:100
Fluence (energy density – mJ/mm²)	6 (low fluence) F= E/spot area	40,000 (high fluence)	1:6,000
Effects	Selective targeting of TM cellular pigment. No thermal or structural damage. Can be repeated.	High absorption by all angle structures, excessive thermal and structural damage. Cannot be repeated. Poor effect in unpigmented TM.	

| Image of tissue damage | 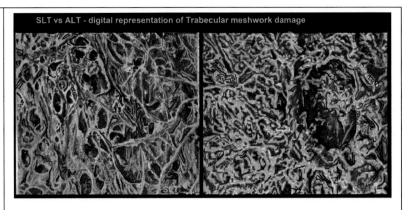 |

Figure 3.15 SLT vs ALT.

ALT is no longer used as it is photo-destructive.
ALT used high energy, long pulse, on a small spot area, causing extremely high energy density, leading to thermal damage of TM and surrounding cells, development of excessive PAS, and angle failure, and could not be repeated.

SLT works with selective thermolysis to improve aqueous drainage, working at lower energy, shorter pulse duration, and lower fluence.

3.6.2 Mechanism of Action

IOP lowering effect of SLT is by increased outflow, which is **immune mediated** (similar to prostaglandin analogue). The effect is described as **selective photo-thermolysis** (intracellular disruption of melanin granules without injuring adjacent cells). **Lack of thermal and structural damage makes SLT repeatable.**

SLT related bio-photoactivation triggers a cytokine response (IL-8, IL-1, TNF) in TM cells, leading to changes in cellular structures and intercellular junctions of TM endothelium (TME) and Schlemm canal endothelium (SCE).

There is an increase in para-cellular spaces and reduced resistance to TM outflow. SLT also triggers a targeted macrophage response to the TM cells, which reactivate the meshwork reducing outflow resistance, improving outflow, and lowering IOP.

SLT can be used with good outcomes in various types of glaucoma. Generally, a higher aqueous inflow and lower outflow are predictive of better response to SLT. This means that the **higher the IOP at presentation, the better the SLT response**. With NTG and conditions that structurally compromise outflow facility, results are less predictable.

- SLT uses low energy (0.3–1.5 mJ), for an extremely short duration (3 nanoseconds), with a large spot (400 µm – pre-set), resulting in low energy density on target tissue. Target tissue is melanin granules within TM cells.
- Precise targeting is not essential; laser is selectively absorbed by intracellular pigment, producing a biological effect stimulating natural mechanisms to enhance aqueous outflow and reduce IOP.

When should SLT be used?

The higher the IOP at presentation, the better the SLT response.
Appropriate patient selection is essential to ensure successful outcome.

Best results	Less effective	Poor outcomes/Avoid
• OHT • POAG • PXF • PDS	• LTG (low tension glaucoma) • Pseudophakic glaucoma • Aphakia • Failed trabeculectomy • Regressed NVG with open angle • CACG with previous PI • Steroid induced glaucoma	• Severe active uveitis • Multiple PAS • Neovascular glaucoma • Patients on long-term steroids • Angle recession glaucoma

SLT response is better, early in the disease spectrum.
- **Early initial treatment with SLT – better, more dramatic response.**
- **Last gasp therapy – modest response or likely to fail** (due to disease progression).

Newly diagnosed OHT and early POAG are ideal patients for SLT.
- **SLT first line therapy** – removes need for topical treatment.
- **SLT second/third line therapy** (in patients with limited response to initial therapy, or with suspect compliance) – improves IOP control, reduces overall number of drops, useful in patients with poor compliance or health issues, used to defer or delay surgical intervention in patients who are not fit for surgery.

How is success defined with SLT treatment?

- **Successful treatment is a >20% IOP REDUCTION, with stable disc and VF, and no further active intervention required.**
- **Success is predicted by baseline IOP but not degree of TM pigmentation**

- **Full effect can take up to 6 months, but trend in response is apparent in 6–8 weeks.**

- **SLT is effective in 75–80% patients. 20–25% will not respond (treatment failure).**

- **Poor response is often due to poor patient selection or sub-optimal laser delivery.**

- SLT improves IOP control without additional medical therapy for 2–5 years. It can be repeated to achieve IOP control for 8–10 years without any topical treatment.

Patient selection is vital for a successful outcome.

Best prognosis	Non-contributory factor	Worse prognosis
High IOP at presentation PXF, PDS, pigmented angle Younger patient (age <60 yr) Treatment naïve eyes (SLT as 1st line treatment)	Age, race, sex, iris colour Refractive errors Angle pigmentation (intracellular pigment is important)	LTG, IOP <20, NAG, PAS, trauma, previous surgery – cataract, trabeculectomy Patient on multiple therapy Advanced glaucoma

Advantages of SLT – simplify treatment in OHT and early POAG.

Avoids side effects associated with topical/ systemic treatments. - No allergies. - No systemic side effects. - No conjunctival scarring – improves filtration surgery outcome.	**More cost-effective** than multiple drops, medical therapy, or surgery. - **Single clinic-based procedure.** - **Medical therapy** – higher costs of drug, nursing care with administration, side-effects. - **Surgery** – higher costs and risks of surgery.

Removes compliance issues associated with drops –100% compliance. Useful in:
- Elderly patients, those who live alone, patients with dementia, drop allergy, arthritis (difficulty with instillation), and to reduce the overall number of drops used.
- Helps defer filtration surgery in poor candidates for surgery.

Prevents IOP fluctuation (peak-trough diurnal fluctuations) associated with drops, with better 24-hour control.

SLT is proven to be as effective as prostaglandin analogues in reducing IOP.

3.6.2.1 Recommendations for SLT Use

SLT as first line Rx – no drops Ideal cohort	SLT as second line Rx (drops + SLT)	SLT as third line Rx (SLT + multiple Rx)
- OHT - Early POAG - Early PXF glaucoma - Pigmentary glaucoma - Elderly patients - Difficulty with drops	- OHT with high IOP - Advanced POAG, PXF or PDS glaucoma - Drop allergy - Compliance issues (*additional drops not desirable*)	- Medical Rx ineffective or inappropriate, ill, elderly patients with no support, arthritis, dementia, poor candidates for surgery
Low risk patients Presenting IOP- 21–30mm Hg with healthy discs. Safe to do SLT (*including waiting + response times*). Patients with IOP >30, with healthy discs, treatment may be started with drops, which can be stopped after SLT.	**High risk patients need more urgent Rx, risk of RVO with high un-Rx IOP.** - More advanced glaucoma needs immediate treatment with drops. - **Drops need to continue after SLT.**	**Advanced glaucoma on maximum medical therapy, or previous failed surgery.** SLT reduces number of drops, helps defer surgery and optimizes IOP control.

High IOP on presentation and early treatment leads to a better response.
Do not perform SLT in patients who have had previous ALT – high risk of complete angle failure with uncontrolled IOP

3.6.3 SLT Laser Technique

Take informed consent, explaining risks/benefits of the procedure.
- Response takes 4–6 months and effects last 2–5 years. It can be repeated if effective the first time. Failure rate is 20–25%, needing other treatment modalities.
- **Patients need to continue with previous glaucoma drops. SLT is in addition to, rather than instead of, drops.**

Pre-treatment
- Patient examination – including IOP check and gonioscopy.
- Pilocarpine 2% (stat dose) is instilled to open the angle.
- Apraclonidine is used to prevent treatment-related IOP spike

Use the Latina Gonio SLT lens with topical anaesthesia and coupling lubricant

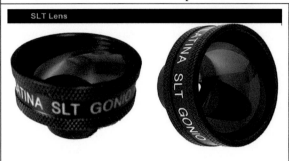

SLT Lens

Latina Gonio SLT lens
Image magnification – ×1.0
Spot magnification – ×1.0
Contact diameter – 14.5mm, tilted anterior lens surface to correct astigmatism and keep laser beam focused. Large 63° mirror for a good angle view (of opposite angle).

SLT is safe and easy to perform but requires expertise at gonioscopy and identifying angle structures. Precise focusing is not important.

Figure 3.16 SLT lens.

Procedure – Switch the laser machine on and select SLT option from the home page.

Slit lamp parameters – adjust:
- IPD, eyepiece refractive error
- Table and chinrest height
- Slit – tallest height, medium width
- Just visible illumination
- Illumination tower is co-axial

SLT laser parameters
- Wavelength – 532 nm
- **Spot size – 400 µm (pre-set)**
- **Pulse duration – 3 ns (pre-set)**
- **Laser energy – 0.6–1.4 mJ**
- **Start with 0.7 mJ**

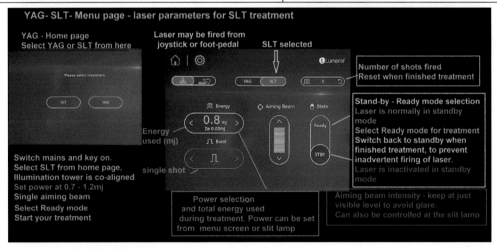

Figure 3.17 YAG SLT menu page.

Power used depends on colour of iris and pigmentation of angle.
- Dark iris and heavily pigmented angle (PDS, PXF) need lower power (**0.4–0.8 mJ**). Treat these patients cautiously (180° of angle at low power).
- **Black – 0.6–1.0 mJ (lower power)**
- **Brown – 0.8–1.2 mJ**
- **Green/blue – 1.0–1.6 mJ (higher power)**

Number of shots – 45–60 per 180 degrees angle. Total number of shots 90–120. Spots are placed adjacent but non-confluent to each other.

- **Always treat 360° for best response (100–120 burns).**
- Exception – **PDS, PXF, heavily pigmented angle – higher inflammatory response, Treat 180°.** *(If initial response is limited, remaining 180° can be treated subsequently.)*

Effective power is achieved when shots generate 1–2 champagne bubbles.
If no bubbles are seen – increase the power by 0.1 mJ.
If excessive bubbles are seen – lower the power by 0.1 mJ.
Ideal power selection is 0.1 mJ lower than the least power that generates 1–2 bubbles.

- Treatment is started with gonioscopy mirror at 12 o'clock position.
- Place aiming spot anywhere in the angle (preferably close to the pigmented TM).
- Aim for discreet, adjacent, non-confluent burns (approximately 25–30 burns/quarter).
- Move sequentially in one direction (generally clockwise). Treat the angle visible in the mirror before rotating the CL and moving to the next quadrant.

Laser burns are not visible with SLT (subthreshold treatment). Identifying treated areas can be difficult, and it is important to keep some anatomical landmark (pigment clump, blood vessel, adjacent iris crypt) in mind, for orientation and to avoid retreating the same areas again.

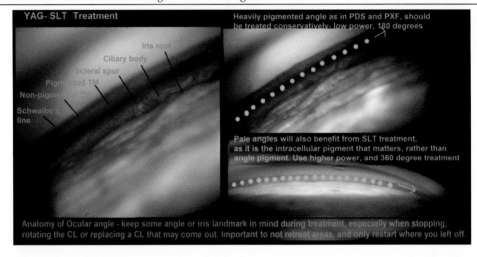

Figure 3.18 YAG SLT treatment.

Post-treatment management
- Apraclonidine (iopidine) is instilled to prevent an IOP spike (5% risk).
- **Steroids dampen the immune mediated SLT effect (cytokine response) and can affect laser outcome**.
  SLT treatment is gentle, without excessive inflammatory response, and steroids are not normally indicated.
- Rarely, a short course (2–3 days) of topical NSAID (Acular) or steroid drops may be given, in PDS or PXF with excessive inflammation.

In summary, SLT can be used as the initial treatment in low-risk glaucoma and OHT, or as adjunct in advanced cases, to control IOP, with good response confirmed by the laser in glaucoma and ocular hypertension (LiGHT) Trial. **SLT can keep low-risk patients under the primary care service in the community, reducing clinic burden.**

3.6.4 Recent Advances

MLT – Micropulse laser trabeculoplasty – MLT uses low energy laser (wavelengths – 532nm, 577nm, or 810nm) in short pulses, with an interval between pulses, allowing cooling, preventing tissue damage, scarring, and inflammation, making it safe, comfortable, and repeatable.

	MLT	SLT	ALT
Wavelength	532, 577, 810 nm	532 nm	488, 514 nm
Spot size	300 μm (useful in narrower angles)	400 μm (large)	50 μm (small)
Mechanism	Photostimulation (no TM cell destruction)	Selective destruction of pigmented TM	Destruction of all angle tissue
Repeatable	Yes	Yes	No, PAS risk
Treatment sign	No visible signs	1–2 champagne bubbles	Visible burns
Post Rx inflam	None	Mild	Severe

SUGGESTED READING

1. Latina, M.A. et al. Q-switched 532-nm Nd:YAG laser trabeculoplasty (SLT): a multicenter, pilot, clinical study. *Ophthalmol.* 1998;105(11): 2082–2088; discussion 2089–2090.

2. Nagar, M. et al. A randomised, prospective study comparing SLT with latanoprost for the control of IOP in OHT and OAG. *Br J Ophthalmol.* 2005;89(11):1413–1417.

3. Melamed, S. et al. SLT as primary treatment for OAG: a prospective, nonrandomized pilot study. *Arch Ophthalmol.* 2003;121(7): 957–960.

4. Gazzard, G. et al. Laser in glaucoma and ocular hypertension (LiGHT) trial. A multicentre, randomised controlled trial: design and methodology. *Br J Ophthalmol.* 2018 May;102(5):593–598.

Section 4 Photothermal Lasers

This chapter aims to improve understanding of photothermal laser machine and techniques to get the ophthalmic trainee started with common retinal treatments, including PRP, sectoral PRP, focal laser treatment, and laser retinopexy.

4.1 INTRODUCTION – TREATMENT CONCEPTS AND CURRENT AND NEW LASER TECHNOLOGY

4.1.1 Current Concepts in Laser Photocoagulation

The advent of the argon laser marked a milestone in retinal photocoagulation. Two large RCTs, Diabetic Retinopathy Study (DRS) and Early Treatment Diabetic Retinopathy Study (ETDRS), confirmed the beneficial effects of early photocoagulation in diabetic retinopathy (reduced moderate vision loss by 50%), and established argon laser as the treatment of choice for diabetic retinopathy.

A variety of photothermal lasers including solid (YAG), gas (argon, krypton), and liquid (tuneable dye), operating in a range of wavelengths – 532 nm (green), 561 nm, 577 nm (yellow), 660 nm (red), and 810 nm (IR) – are in use. Slit lamp mounted lasers have improved delivery. Endo-lasers using fibre-optic probes have shortened treatment time and improved results in VR surgery.

Argon Laser
CW laser, emitting 2 wavelengths, 488 nm (blue) and 514 nm (green) light. **Blue light is preferentially absorbed by macular pigments, with a high risk of macular burns, and not safe for treatment. Green wavelength works on RPE melanin and is used for PRP and FLT, with single spot (size 100–500 μm) and long pulse (100–200 ms),** which makes argon slow, painful, and more photo-destructive. They have been replaced by newer lasers.

Krypton Laser
CW laser emitting 647 nm (red) and 568 nm (yellow) wavelengths. Red wavelength is not absorbed by luteal pigments but is more damaging due to deeper choroidal penetration. Krypton yellow is similar to the yellow dye laser, which is more readily available.

Dye Laser
Provides a wide range of wavelengths (green, yellow, red 570–630 nm). Green and red have no advantages over argon and krypton respectively, with similar side-effects. **Yellow wavelength (577 nm) is absorbed by haemoglobin, allowing treatment of mA and blood vessels with lower power, useful in patients with a thin retina or low pain threshold.**

Diode Laser and SDM (Subthreshold Diode Micro-pulse) Laser
Compact, portable laser, working at 810 nm (IR wavelength), for PRP, PDT for vascular AMD, treatment of small choroidal melanoma by transpupillary thermotherapy (TTT), and cyclo-diode. It has deeper penetration (90% absorbed by choroidal melanocytes), works safely through a haemorrhage (not absorbed by blood), and penetrates sclera for trans-scleral treatment in presence of media opacities (cyclo-diode).
SDM laser selectively targets RPE and choroidal melanin, with extremely short pulses (100us) with recovery intervals between pulses (1900us), reducing pain and outer retinal damage, thereby maintaining retinal function and structural integrity.

KTP Frequency-doubled Neodymium-Yttrium Aluminium Garnet (Nd-YAG) Laser
YAG emits 1064 nm (IR) wavelength but can be made to emit at second harmonic (frequency doubling) using a KTP crystal, at 532 nm (green), which is absorbed by melanin for retinal treatment. The pulse duration of the KTP frequency doubled YAG laser is shorter (10–30 ms), making it safer, more comfortable, and less photo-destructive than an argon laser.

PASCAL laser (PAttern SCAn Laser)
is a class 4, frequency doubled OPSL (optically pumped semiconductor solid laser) that offers multi-spot treatment, reducing treatment times and risk of phototoxicity.

The previous concept of **photo-destruction considered visible burns to be effective treatment.** It stabilized the underlying condition but caused significant morbidity from collateral damage, with reduced acuity, contrast sensitivity, night vision, paracentral and peripheral field loss, exacerbation of DME, distortion of retinal anatomy with tractional bands, macular pucker, and retinal folds, significantly affecting functional visual outcomes, ability to drive, and QoL.

4.1.2 New Laser Treatments/Technology

Ideal photo-coagulative treatment achieves therapeutic benefits while preserving visual function, without causing retinal damage.

New concepts in photocoagulation include altering laser parameters to reduce retinal damage and improving delivery efficiency, accuracy, and safety.

4.1.2.1 Reduce Retinal Damage

Retinal preservation and restoration of function is achieved by:
Use of small spots – uses less energy, causing smaller scars. (Use 200 μm spot for PRP and 100 μm spot size for FLT.) Use of large spots should be abandoned.
Increased inter-spot gap – preserves retina between burns. Previous use of heavy, confluent burns is no longer acceptable.
Reduced pulse duration – a CW laser (argon) causes more thermal injury. A **laser pulse can be reduced to milliseconds (PASCAL), microseconds (MPL – micro-pulse laser), and nanoseconds (NPL),** making treatment more comfortable and less damaging. A shorter pulse duration reduces heat dissipation and collateral damage of the inner retina.
Use of longer wavelengths – yellow and IR wavelengths have better penetration and are less damaging. IR wavelength is not absorbed by blood, making it safer to use in the presence of retinal or vitreous haemorrhages.
Use of subthreshold power that does not cause visible burns (EPM, SLT).
Combining all above – short pulse + long wavelength + low power – EPM, SDL.
Quicker delivery and faster treatments – using pattern delivery modes with pattern and navigated lasers.

Conventional lasers are destructive, working on the principle of overt thermal damage to leaking blood vessels, creating oxygen bridges, reducing hypoxia by lowering oxygen demand, and decreasing retinal metabolic rate. The beneficial effects are offset by significant visual side-effects and disruption of retinal anatomy through scarring.

The current concept in modern retinal laser therapy (MRT) is one of photo-stimulation rather than photo-destruction.

Photo-stimulation maintains vision by **slow onset, but longer-lasting benefits**. The temperature achieved in the retina does not cause cell death, only damage to organelles, which undergo repair with over-expression of multiple genes that alter retinal physiology and metabolism, and promote mitochondrial activation and cellular proliferation to initiate repair and healing. Therapeutic effects are mediated physiologically by altering the cytokine-led immune pathway, downregulation of VEGF and PEDF, and acceleration of RPE heat shock protein (HSP) in dysfunctional cells, restoring normality.

4.1.2.2 Principles of Modern Retinal Laser Therapy (MRT)

Therapeutic effects are from **thermal stress** (cells affected but not killed). MRT is effective without causing visible burns.
Treating larger areas of dysfunctional retina with subthreshold energy amplifies the cellular response, optimizes therapeutic effects, and improves efficacy of MRT. **MRT works on the principle of high density–low intensity treatment.**
MRT considers maculopathy to be a spectrum of retinopathy, and aims to treat all areas of dysfunctional retina, extending beyond the macula for maximum benefit. (FLT is not a concept of MRT.) **There is no need to specifically target microaneurysms as mechanism of action does not involve thermal photocoagulation.**
MRT is non-destructive and non-inflammatory, leading to better outcomes. Higher power does not improve therapeutic benefits, only risk of damage.
MRT is repeatable and effective for trans foveal treatment with FLT and PRP in DR, RVO, CSCR, RAM, and other retinal vasculopathies.

Shorter Pulse Lasers
A continuous wave (CW) laser (argon, krypton) has a pulse duration of 50–200 ms causing visible burns and retinal damage.
Reducing pulse duration reduces heat dissipation, causing less thermal damage
Milli-pulse Laser **PASCAL** (milli-pulse laser) has a pulse duration of 10–30 ms, which is 5–6 times less than argon, resulting in lower photothermal injury.
PASCAL EPM (end-point management = millisecond pulse + subthreshold power) EPM uses millisecond pulse with low power (**30% of normal threshold power)** to treat all dysfunctional retinal areas (high-density treatment to entire posterior pole, except the central FAZ). The clinical effect is achieved without any visible burns (either clinically, or with fundal imaging – OCT, FAF, FFA). Treatment can be repeated in 3 months.

Micro-pulse Laser (MPL) – Iridex MPL System

MPL shortens pulse duration to extremely short repetitive pulses of 0.1–0.5 us (short 'on' time) with intervals between pulses (long 'off' time). The off time allows tissue cooling between treatments, preventing heat dissipation to surrounding tissues. The ratio between on and off times is called the duty cycle, usually 5% with MRT.

Multiple lasers offer MPL capability. It can be used with IR (810 nm), yellow (577 nm), and green (532 nm) wavelengths. MPL lasers are primarily used for treating macular diseases because they selectively target RPE, while sparing the surrounding neurosensory retina.

Subthreshold MPL promotes retinal healing with a restorative effect on RPE function, and may re-sensitize RPE in wet AMD, which is unresponsive to anti-VEGF therapy. MPL can be used in retinal diseases and glaucoma (MLT-micro-pulse laser trabeculoplasty).

MPL in DME has provided valuable insight into laser mechanism, **demonstrating that direct closure of microaneurysms with heavy burn is not necessary to achieve therapeutic results.**

Nano-pulse Laser (NPL)

Retina regeneration therapy (2RT; Ellex) is a subthreshold nano-pulse laser using a 532 nm laser to produce 3 ns pulses, which are postulated to stimulate renewal of RPE and have shown promising results in slowing progression of AMD and improving sensitivity to anti-VEGF response.

4.1.2.3 Concept of Subthreshold Laser Treatment

The term 'sub-threshold' refers to photocoagulation that does not produce visible burns, either by examination or standard imaging modalities. It is also called **non damaging retinal treatment (NRT).** Subthreshold effects can be attained by reducing laser power. Electron microscopy has shown that 10–25% of visible threshold power will affect RPE, while sparing the overlying retina.

A major disadvantage of the subthreshold laser is **lack of reliable titration to achieve reproducible sub-visible treatment, leading to variability in treatment**. If the laser settings are too low, treatment will be sub-therapeutic; if too high, excessive retinal damage is a risk, especially with the high-density perifoveal coverage.

High-density macular coverage with relatively small spots is time-consuming, difficult to monitor, with no visible scars (to avoid re-treatment). PASCAL EPM overcomes this by delivering a pre-set pattern with a few visible marker burns.

There is a risk of undertreatment (because not enough 'area' has been treated), and it may be difficult to ascertain if lack of improvement is from undertreatment or poor response. Detailed documentation of treated areas is vital to plan the next course of action. However, one concept is that, as treatment is subthreshold and non-damaging, it can be repeated, even in previously treated areas, making the above concern irrelevant.

4.1.2.4 Subthreshold Diode Micro-pulse (SDM) Laser

SDM, a **micro-pulse** diode laser (**MPL + subthreshold power + longer wavelength**), is absorbed selectively by RPE, causing sublethal effects. The low-intensity effect is amplified by placement of confluent laser spots (high-density treatment) over the entire area of retinal pathology. SDM works by normalizing RPE function and can be used alone or in combination with drug therapy to achieve retina-sparing disease management.

4.1.2.5 New Laser Delivery Systems

New delivery systems speed up treatment in a controlled, efficient, and safe manner.

In traditional laser delivery with slit lamp – CL system – viewing, locating, and accurately targeting all microaneurysms can be difficult. Microaneurysms are not always clinically visible, and dependent on media clarity and user experience.

4.1.2.6 Navilas Laser System

NAVILAS uses **computer-guided eye tracking** (retinal navigation), integrated with **fundus camera-based delivery** (not slit lamp-contact lens delivery). The 532 nm (green) laser integrates fundus imaging (FFA or red-free images can be overlaid on a fundal photo to precisely map and target mA, and plan treatment areas). Eye tracking enhances safety, precision, and accuracy of laser delivery, which is monitored on a screen. The field of view is 50° for FLT, and 80° for PRP, and both treatments can be performed using retinal eye tracking, with 96% accuracy in FLT, using grid patterns (TREX-DME trial). A newer model uses 577nm wavelength (yellow) laser and combines **navigation with subthreshold (MPL) laser** delivery.

Navigated lasers are limited by the learning curve, higher cost, and need for FFA in every patient. In addition, MRT negates the concept of targeting mA.

4.1.2.7 Multi-spot Pattern Laser Systems

Many lasers offer predetermined pattern delivery with standardized spot size and inter spot distance, making PRP quicker, less painful, and more effective.

PASCAL – Topcon Lumenis – Array Laser link Navilas	Nidek (Fremont, CA) Ellex's (Minneapolis, MN) Rapide model	Quantel Medical (Bozeman, MT) The Supra Scan laser Iridex

MRT is non-damaging, potentially repeatable, and maintains visual function (VA, colour vision, contrast sensitivity, and VF) better. There is reduced risk of scarring, pigmentary changes, CNV, scotomas, subretinal fibrosis, RPE atrophy or choroidal hypoperfusion.

4.1.2.8 Use of Selective and Targeted Retinal Therapy

Selective Retinal Therapy (SRT) is a subthreshold approach using MPL or NPL to selectively target RPE cells, while preserving photoreceptors and neural retina. The surrounding healthy cells proliferate and migrate into treated areas, improving metabolism of diseased retina and aiding healing.

Targeted retinal photocoagulation (TRP) – subthreshold laser therapy aimed at specific target. Examples are FLT in DME, feeder vessel photocoagulation in CNV, or PRP in areas of peripheral ischaemia identified with wide-field fluorescein angiography.

SUGGESTED READING

1. Luttrull, J.K. et al. SDM laser as invisible retinal phototherapy for DME: review. *Curr Diabetes Rev.* 2012;8:274–284.

2. Sivaprasad, S. et al. SDM laser therapy: evolution and clinical applications. *Surv Ophthalmol.* 2010;55:516–530.

3. Nagpal, M. Comparison of laser photocoagulation for diabetic retinopathy using 532-nm standard laser versus multispot pattern scan laser. *Retina.* 2010;30:452–458.

4. Chappelow, A.V. et al. PRP for PDR: pattern scan laser versus argon laser. *Am J Ophthalmol.* 2012;153:780–781.

5. Kernt, M. et al. FLT and PRP with a navigated laser (NAVILAS). *Acta Ophthalmol.* 2011;89:662–664.

6. Lavinsky, D. et al. Randomized clinical trial evaluating mETDRS versus normal or high-density micropulse photocoagulation for DME. *Invest Ophthalmol Vis Sci.* 2011;52:4314–4323.

7. Blumenkranz, M.S. et al. Semiautomated PASCAL for retinal photocoagulation. *Retina.* 2006;26:370–376.

8. Chablani, J. et al. Restorative retinal laser therapy: present state and future direction. *Surv Ophth.* 2018;63:307–328.

9. Majcher, C. et al. A review of micropulse laser photocoagulation. *Rev of Optometry.* 2011; Nov:10–17.

4.2 GETTING STARTED WITH LASER RETINAL PHOTOCOAGULATION

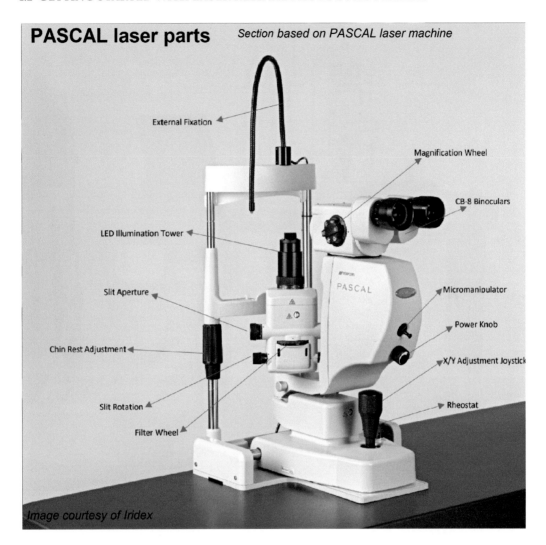

Figure 4.1 Parts of laser – PASCAL.

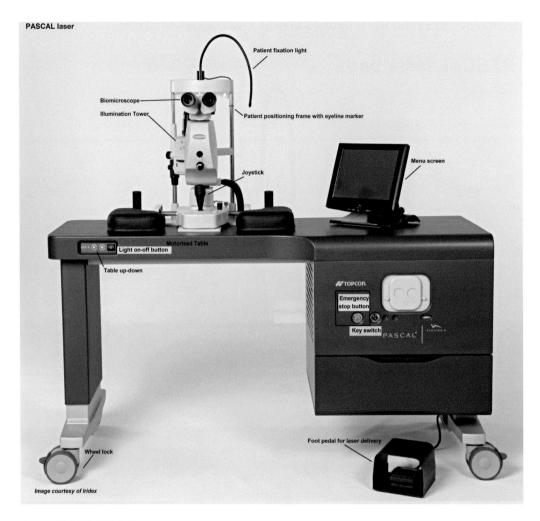

Figure 4.2 PASCAL laser.

4.2.1 PASCAL Laser Machine

The PASCAL laser is a class 4, frequency doubled, optically pumped semiconductor (solid) laser, emitting 532 (green) or 577 (yellow) wavelengths, designed to treat retinal vascular diseases. It can be used with a slit-lamp or indirect ophthalmoscope, using a single or variety of predetermined multi-spot patterns, for quick, efficient delivery of short millisecond pulses.

Slit lamp is standard, with a housing **key switch, emergency stop button, on/off button, table up and down button, menu screen, and viewer screen.**

Slit lamp adjustments – set
• Table height, chin rest, eyepiece IPD, and refractive errors.
• **Magnification – ×6 to view and perform PRP**. • **Increase magnification to ×10 or ×16 for FLT**.
• **Just visible slit illumination.** Excessive light causes glare, blanching of aiming beam, and risk of phototoxicity with prolonged treatment time.
• **Maximum slit height** (no further adjustments required).
• **Medium slit width** to allow a reasonable fundal view. • **Narrowing the beam – decreases field of view (FOV) but increases depth of focus**. Narrow beams sharpen focus and allow better view of subtle details like mA. • However, **do not make the beam so narrow that you lose your retinal bearings.** Beam width must allow adequate FOV, **keeping the fovea and disc in view.**

The menu screen is used to select laser treatment parameters and aiming beam intensity.

The 3-D controller (on older machines) can be used to adjust laser parameters and manipulate patterns, power settings, and laser position but are fiddly to use, and not essential for treatment. It is recommended that you adjust your settings via the touch screen.

Getting Started

Switching on – switch on the mains and turn the key. Wait for the laser to boot up.

- Display screen shows anterior or posterior treatment (**home page**).

- Select **posterior treatment for retinal phototherapy.**
- Select **anterior treatment for PSLT.**

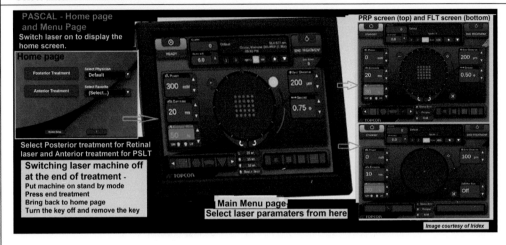

Figure 4.3 PASCAL home page and menu page – 1.

- **Always keep the laser in stand-by mode.**
- **Only activate (ready mode) when ready to treat.**

Switching off – once treatment is complete

- Place system back in standby mode (A). Press END TREATMENT (F) on screen.

- Return to the home page. Turn off the key switch. Wait for the machine to shut down.

- Remove key and hand it to a named nurse.

DO NOT USE THE EMERGENCY BUTTON TO SHUT OFF THE LASER – this de-activates the key switch. Only use emergency button in a genuine emergency.

- **If the emergency button has been activated, it needs to be pressed again to deactivate it, to allow the key switch to function normally.**

Posterior Treatment Display Screen

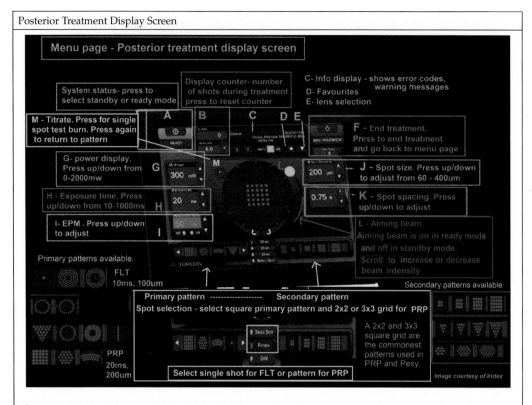

Figure 4.4 Menu screen – posterior segment display page – 2.

Switch on the laser, and select posterior treatment.

Select the pattern for PRP and retinopexy – multiple options are available, but a 2×2 and 3×3 square grid are commonest used. The machine autoselects spot size (200 μm) and pulse duration (20ms). Other patterns, although available, do not add any further value to your treatment.
Set power and select ready mode for treatment, delivered using the foot pedal.

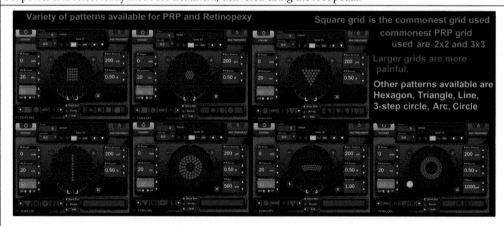

Figure 4.5 Variety of patterns for PRP and Retinopexy – 1.

Select single spot for FLT – the machine autoselects 100 μm spot size and 10 ms pulse duration.
Macular grid patterns – although available, are not used except with EPM. Single shots represent a more controlled method of FLT.
Set power and select ready for treatment.

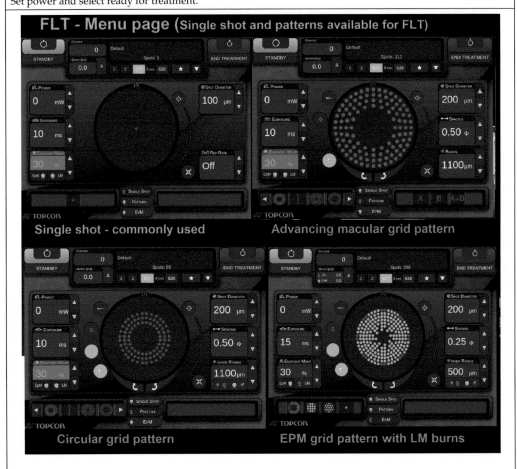

Figure 4.6 Patterns for FLT.

4.2.1.1 Laser Treatment Parameters

	FLT	PRP, retinopexy
	Select single shot	Select pattern
Spot size	100 μm (range from 50–200 μm) 50 μm for mA close to FAZ	200 μm (range from 200–400 μm) Do not use larger spots
Pulse duration	10 ms (range from 10–20 ms) Use 15–20 ms if poor reaction	20 ms (range from 20–40 ms) Use 25–30 ms if poor reaction
Spot space	NA	1–1.5 (for PRP); 0 for retinopexy
Power	100–250 mw	250–500 mw
Pattern	NA	Square pattern 3×3 and 2×2 for PRP 2×2 for retinopexy
Reaction	Light grey burn	Light white burn – PRP Deep white burn – retinopexy

- **Select threshold power – least power for just visible burn,** by **titration in a safe area.**
- Inexperienced users should not exceed 200 mw for FLT and 500 mw for PRP.
- Patients with media opacities, vitreous haemorrhage, and pale retinas require higher power to be effective. Use lower power in aphakia, pseudophakia, and pigmented fundi.
- **Reduce power if you reduce the spot size.**

Documentation of Laser Treatment on Completion
- **Number of shots × pulse duration × spot size × power used × lens used.**
- Document range of power, spot size, or pulse duration, if it was altered during treatment.

Troubleshooting

What if you cannot see the aiming beam?
If aiming beam is not visible – do the following in order. Ensure:
- Laser is not on stand-by mode.
- Focus is optimal, and CL is not tilted.
- Reduce slit lamp illumination slightly (aiming beam easier to see).
- Increase aiming beam intensity slightly.

What if you cannot see laser burns?
With appropriate titration and laser parameters, a light grey burn for FLT and a light white burn for PRP is visible during treatment. Inability to see burns is due to:
- Poor slit lamp focus, including slit width and magnification.
- Patient movement.
- Wrong lens, tilting CL, air bubbles.
- Low power selection.
- Glare from slit lamp or aiming beam.
- Media opacity – corneal scar, cataract, poor dilation, corneal abrasion.

Increasing power with poor visibility is not advisable, as it increases laser hazards and causes painful treatment. Address in the following sequence – improve focus, then adjust power, and lastly adjust pulse duration.

Seeing burns better – burns may be present but are not visible due to poor view. - Improve slit lamp focus, including eyepiece. - Reduce glare (adjust illumination). - Narrow slit slightly to increase depth of focus. - Ensure CL is flat; avoid tilting, excessive manipulation, air bubbles, corneal erosions. - **Change CL to one that offers better magnification.** Mainster ×1 or a 3-mirror lens offer better view of the retina and burns (wide-field lenses minify the view). - Increase slit lamp magnification, to improve titration and establish treatment power, then complete PRP at lower magnification. (**High magnification reduces FOV and can cause loss of orientation.**)	**If burns are still not visible**, it may be due to a pale retina, media opacities, or suboptimal laser parameter selection. - **Increase power** (if patient tolerates it). - **Increase exposure time** (25–30 ms). - **Reduce spot size and power accordingly.** - Seek nursing help with difficult patients. - Ensure slit lamp is serviced regularly.

4.3 PAN RETINAL PHOTOCOAGULATION

Pan retinal photocoagulation is standard treatment for retinal vascular diseases, including the 2 common conditions, PDR and CRVO. The efficacy and benefits of PRP have been established by DRS and ETDRS studies. PRP reduces the risk of severe visual loss by 50%.

PRP can be used alone or in conjunction with medical therapy or surgical interventions. Retinal ischaemia provides the neovascular drive, and PRP involves treating large portions of ischaemic retina, with photothermal laser, to reduce hypoxia, reverse ischaemic drive, and stabilize the vascular condition.

Visible and IR wavelengths used in PRP are absorbed by melanin in RPE and choroid, and blood haemoglobin, raising retinal temperature, resulting in protein denaturation, with typical white retinal burn. The extent of damage is related to laser energy and pulse duration used during treatment.

As discussed previously, the main problem with photothermal lasers is the associated damage to overlying neurosensory retina from heat diffusion. This damage is inevitable with current lasers, and tends to be severe with use of excessive power, long pulses, and large spots, resulting in painful treatment and visual loss, limiting the benefits of treatment.

Current photothermal lasers do not improve vision. They essentially stabilize the vascular disease and maintain vision. With progression of vascular disease and use of more laser treatment, visual loss is inevitable.

Photo-destruction results in excessive scarring with poor visual outcome, compromising the patient's ability to drive, affecting their livelihood, independence, and confidence.

It is essential to maintain maximum visual function, including VA, VF, contrast sensitivity, colour vision, and dark-light adaptation for as long as possible. With this goal in mind, treatment concepts have shifted from photo-destruction to using gentle treatment with low power, small spots, and short pulse, to reduce structural damage and preserve function.

4.3.1 Methods of PRP Delivery

Slit lamp – CL delivery is the commonest route for PRP, allowing safe, controlled delivery, with standardized spot size and optimal spot spacing, in all parts of the retina, including the posterior pole. It offers better control over areas to treat or avoid and better titration to select threshold energy, for safer, more comfortable treatment. Additionally, contact lenses prevent blinking, stabilize the eye, and magnify the view in comparison to LIO.

Laser Indirect Ophthalmoscopy (LIO) delivery uses a non-contact condensing lens (20D with well dilated pupil or 28D with small pupil) to focus the laser on the retina.

LIO offers a larger FOV and better access to anterior retina, using scleral indentation. It can be administered with patients lying down in theatre under sedation or GA, useful in anxious patients with a low pain threshold. The disadvantages are a minified view, non-standardized spot (size varies with movement close to or away from patient), and difficulty treating the posterior pole in a safe and controlled manner.

Laser can also be delivered by:

Trans-scleral route

Endolaser – using fibre-optic probe, during vitrectomy.

Navilas uses a fundal camera system for laser delivery.

4.3.2 Normal Ocular Anatomy

Clarity on retinal anatomy and visual function is important for safe, appropriate laser delivery.

• **Diameter of adult eye – 21–27 mm.** • Emmetropic eye is approximately 24.2 mm transverse/ horizontal axis, 23.7 mm sagittal/vertical axis, and 22.0–24.8 mm axial/ ant-post axis. Circumferential diameter of adult eye • at equator is 69–72 mm. • at ora is 50–60 mm.	The eye consists of • **Outer layer** of sclera and cornea. • **Middle layer** of choroid, ciliary body, and iris. • **Inner layer** of retina, extends 360° circumferentially, from optic nerve to the ora serrata anteriorly. • Total area of the retina is approximately 1,100 mm². • The ora serrata lies 6–8 mm behind the limbus. • Nasal ora is narrow (0.8 mm) and 6 mm behind the limbus; the temporal ora is wide (2.1 mm wide) and 8mm behind the limbus.

• Precise measurement of optic disc diameter and disc-to-fovea distance is essential for correlation of topographic and clinical information.
• The retina is transparent up to RPE – **neurosensory retina** (except BV).
• It appears orange, due to the background of the blood-filled choroidal layer.
• The retina is studied using fundal photography, FAF, FFA, laser polarimetry, OCT, and OCT-A.

The average thickness of a healthy retina is:
• 250 µm adjacent to the optic nerve.
• **400 µm in the macular area** around the fovea (para fovea).
• 100–150 µm in the foveola.
• The peripheral retina is thin (beyond equatorial region) – 80 µm at the ora serrata.

The retina has dual circulation.
• The outer retina (outer plexiform – choroid) is nourished by branches of posterior ciliary arteries.
• The inner retina is supplied by branches of the central retinal artery.
• Macular vessels arise from branches of ST and IT arteries.
• **There is a capillary-free avascular zone of approximately 500 µm in the fovea (FAZ).**
• **The fovea forms the anatomical centre of the retina.**
• Approximately 20% people have dual macular circulation (CRA and cilioretinal arteries).
• **Retinal blood vessels are non-fenestrated and maintain the blood-retinal barrier.** (Choroidal vessels are fenestrated.)
• Arterial branches supply capillary networks, draining into venules and the central retinal vein.
• The arterial circulation emanating from the posterior ciliary arteries drains out via 1 or 2 vortex veins in each quadrant, which merge into the ophthalmic vein.
• The optic nerve is located 4.5–5 mm nasal to the fovea with no overlying retinal tissue, causing a blind spot. In the adult eye, the optic disc has an average diameter of 1.86 ± 0.21 mm vertically, and 1.75 ± 0.19 mm horizontally.

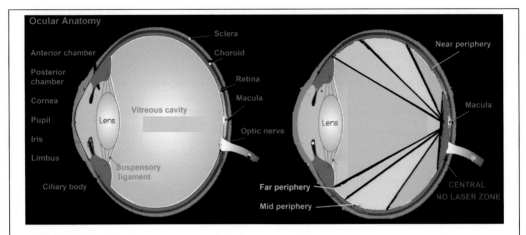

Figure 4.7 Ocular anatomy.

For PRP laser treatment, the retina is divided into three zones – near, mid, and far periphery.

Macula Lutea
- **The macula is the anatomical centre of the retina** (represents 0° on 180° axis).
- **It is 5.5 mm (3.5DD) in diameter, elliptical, and contributes to the central 18° of VF.**
- The centre of the macula is approximately 3.42 ± 0.34 mm temporal and slightly inferior to the temporal margin of the optic disc.
- Foveal cells have a **yellowish appearance due to the presence of xanthophyll and beta carotenoid pigment – lutein and zeaxanthin in the outer plexiform layer. These pigments protect cones from high intensity blue light**.
- **Fovea centralis** – centre of macula, responsible for highest level of visual acuity, colour vision, and brightness perception. It is 100µm thick, with the densest concentration of cones and an absence of rods. It is 1.5 mm (1DD) in size, with a central pit called foveola (0.35 mm), and contributes to the central 5° of visual field.
- **Parafovea** – a 2.5 mm area around the fovea centralis, with a high density of cones and more than five layers of ganglion cells, with a one-to-one correspondence with photoreceptors.
- **Perifovea** – 1.5 mm area around parafovea, with few cones and 2–4 ganglion cell layers.
- **Foveal avascular zone** – is the central 0.5 mm (500 µm) area with no blood vessels.

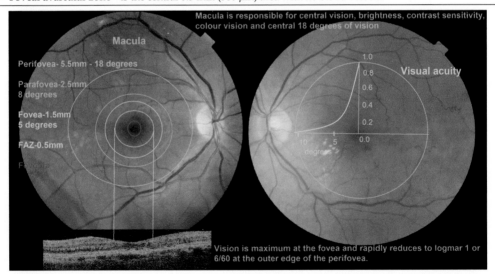

Figure 4.8 Macular parts and function.

Understanding Visual Function

The macula provides:
- **Maximum central vision, colour vision, brightness perception, contrast sensitivity.**
- **Central 18° of VF.**

VA is maximum at the fovea, and rapidly reduces to logMAR 1 or 6/60 at the outer edge of the perifovea.

The remaining retina provides the field of vision (FOV). Each retinal quadrant provides VF in the diametrically opposite area.
Inferior retina – provides superior VF. Superior VF is not vital for functional vision, so the inferior retina can be treated early during PRP.
Superior retina – provides inferior VF. Inferior VF is useful for reading and vision going down the stairs. Superior retina should be treated sparingly with PRP to begin with.
Temporal retina – provides nasal VF. The temporal retina tends to be most ischaemic, more likely to develop NV, especially in the watershed zone (temporal to macula), and **should be treated early and actively with PRP.**
Nasal retina – provides temporal VF. Temporal VF is important for driving vision, and should be spared for as long as possible.
The central 30° and the nasal 30° of the near periphery together account for 60° of driving vision. This area should be spared for as long as possible when doing PRP.

4.3.2.1 Indication for Pan Retinal Photocoagulation

- Severe NPDR in high-risk patients.

- Proliferative DR.

- Ischaemic CRVO.

- Radiation retinopathy.

- Ocular ischaemic syndrome (suspect carotid artery stenosis, with asymmetric retinopathy).

- Early neovascular glaucoma.

- Exudative retinal vascular disorders – sickle cell retinopathy, retinal telangiectasia, Coat's disease, and retinal capillary haemangioma.

- Peripheral retinal ischaemic retinopathies – familial exudative vitreoretinopathy, vasculitis, and retinopathy of prematurity.

- Tumours – vaso-proliferative retinal tumours, angiomas. Laser photocoagulation can promote closure of feeder blood vessels.

4.3.3 How Does PRP Work?

Effective photocoagulation targets retinal pigments – melanin and haemoglobin.

- Melanin absorbs green, yellow, red, and infrared wavelengths.

- Haemoglobin absorbs blue, green, and yellow, but not red wavelength.

In simplistic terms, PRP sacrifices the peripheral ischaemic retina to stabilize the vascular disease and maintain the central vision.

A well done PRP targets mid and far peripheral retina, with barely visible laser burns. Laser energy absorbed by RPE raises the retinal temperature. Temperature > 65°C causes coagulation necrosis with denaturation of cellular proteins, making the clear retina opaque at the burn site (white burn).

- Destruction of ischaemic retina reduces production of angiogenic factors, while the remaining healthy retina produces anti-angiogenic factors, altering the angiogenic drive.

- RPE and photoreceptors are high oxygen utilizing cells, and their selective destruction increases oxygen availability to the remaining retina, reducing hypoxia.

- Destruction of RPE, creates direct oxygen bridges from choroid to the inner retina, improving oxygenation.

- Laser induced PVD promotes new vessel involution and lowers the risk of vitreous haemorrhage.

- **PRP reduces risk of PDR to 4% and the need for PPV (vitrectomy) by 50%.**

The treatment plan varies with disease presentation and severity. The natural endpoint of treatment is the regression of proliferative changes and stabilization of underlying disease. The overall regression rates are 67–75% for mild–moderate PDR and 43% (40–45%) in severe PDR.

A recent study, Protocol S of Diabetic Retinopathy Clinical Research Network (DRCR. net), found that anti-VEGF monotherapy for PDR is as effective as PRP. However, anti-VEGF therapy requires multiple injections, and long-term commitment (socio-economic consider-ations), making it an unviable option. Laser PRP therefore remains the current mainstay treatment for retinal vascular diseases.

4.3.4 Getting Started with Pan Retinal Photocoagulation

An understanding of retinal anatomy and disease pathology is important to perform a safe PRP. The technique is as important as the treatment plan, and understanding who to treat, when, why, how much, and when to stop or consider alternative treatment options, is vital. (*Some prior clinical experience in retinal pathology and handling CL is useful prior to PRP.*)

- The macula is the anatomical centre of the retina (represents 0° on a horizontal or vertical meridian extending from ora to ora).
- The retina extends 90° on each side, above and below the macula.
- The optic nerve lies approximately 20° nasal to the macula.
- 1DD (disc diameter) = 1.5 mm, represents approximately 5 degrees.

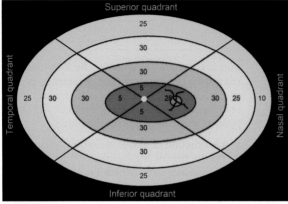
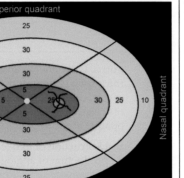

The four zones are
- **Central red zone** – 5° superior, inferior, temporal, and 25° nasal. **No laser done in this zone.**
- **Near periphery (green) zone** – 30° around central zone. Spare this zone for as long as possible, to preserve driving vision.
- **Mid periphery (yellow) zone** – 30° superior, inferior and temporal and 25° nasal. Treat this area actively and early (most ischaemic).
- **Far periphery (lilac) zone** – 25° superior, inferior and temporal and 10° nasal. Treat actively; peripheral ischaemia contributes to persistent disease activity.

Figure 4.9 Getting started with PRP – 1.

Divide retina into 4 zones and 4 quadrants, centred at the fovea.
Four quadrants are: superior, inferior, nasal, and temporal.

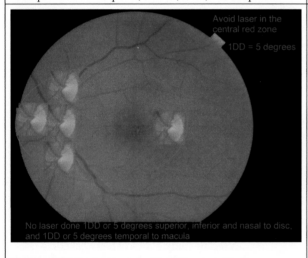

- **The central red zone should not be lasered during PRP treatment (includes disc and macula).**
- It provides central 30° of VF (5 degrees temporal and 25° nasal to fovea).
- 1 DD = 5 degrees.
- Avoid 1DD superior, inferior and nasal to the optic disc, and 1DD temporal to the macula.

The remaining retina is available for PRP (equates to 85° inferior, superior and temporal, and 65° nasal quadrant).

Figure 4.10 Getting started with PRP – central red zone.

The **near peripheral zone** (surrounding 30°) should be spared for as long as possible. **The red and green zones together give 60° VF, which is vital for driving.**

The **mid-peripheral zone** extending up to the equator **tends to be most ischaemic, requiring early and active PRP treatment.**

The **far periphery** extends from the equator to the ora serrata.

Zones	Quadrants			
	Superior	Inferior	Temporal	Nasal
Central red zone	5	5	5	25
Near periphery – green	30	30	30	30
Mid-periphery – yellow	30	30	30	25
Far periphery – lilac	25	25	25	10

4.3.5 Schematic Approach to PRP

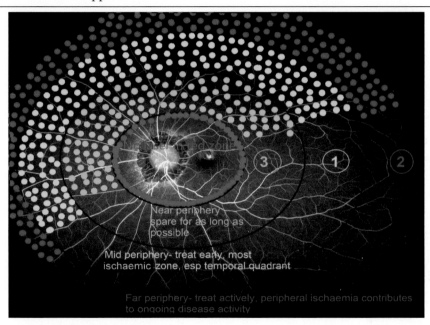

Figure 4.11 Schematic approach to PRP.

First-Line Treatment – Mid-peripheral Retina (Yellow Zone)
- Always start PRP in mid-periphery – most ischaemic area.
- **Start treatment in inferior quadrant** – safe area to treat (superior VF not vital for function), and reduces risk of lost opportunity from future vitreous haemorrhage.
- **Treat superior retina next** (does not affect driving VF)
- **Treat temporal quadrant actively**, especially the watershed area (temporal to the macula tends to be ischaemic with risk of developing NVE).
- **Treat nasal quadrant sparingly** for as long as possible – to preserve driving VF.
- **Order of PRP in mid-periphery is inferior–superior–temporal–nasal.**
- **Always keep 1–1.5 spot gap between burns to preserve peripheral VF.**

Second-Line Treatment – Far Peripheral Retina (Purple Zone)
- If disease remains active, the next zone to treat is the far periphery.
- Peripheral ischaemia contributes to persistent DME and proliferative activity.
- All four quadrants can be safely treated, as visual function is not affected.
- There is less risk of PRP-induced DME when treating this quadrant.

Third-Line Treatment – Near Peripheral Retina (Green Zone)
- PRP in this zone will affect driving VF, so treatment is only reserved for ongoing activity with florid neovascularization.
- **Treat sparingly with larger gaps to preserve VF as much as possible.**

Common Mistakes Made during PRP
- **To spare temporal retina**, due to macula being present in this quadrant. This area tends to be ischaemic (CWS, dark haemorrhages, IRMA, NVE) and needs active, early treatment.
- **To treat nasal quadrant with extensive laser**, as it is perceived as a safer quadrant. Nasal retina provides temporal VF, which is important for driving, and should be treated sparingly.

Pre-PRP investigations – allow objective measurements of retinal vascular disease, monitor prevalence, severity, and help in decision-making for treatment and prognosis.

FFA – useful in identifying IRMA and neovascularization, and extent of mid-peripheral capillary dropout in ischaemic patients, but misses ischaemia in the far periphery.

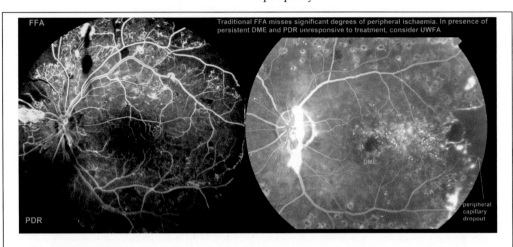

Figure 4.12 FFA in PRP – 1.

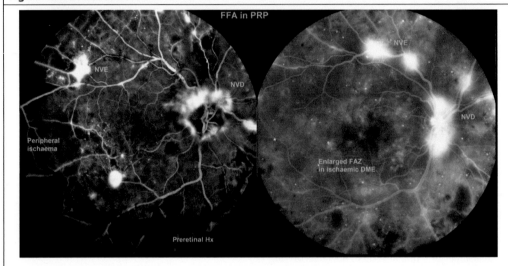

Figure 4.13 FFA in PRP – 2.

Ultra-widefield FFA (UWFA)

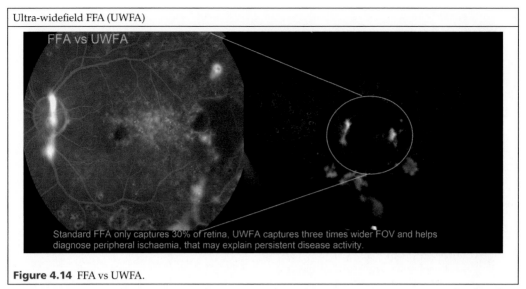

Figure 4.14 FFA vs UWFA.

Identification of peripheral non-perfused areas, and calculation of ischaemic index using UWFA, correlates with disease severity and progression (fourfold increase in progression to PDR and DME). Peripheral non-perfusion is an independent risk factor for DME incidence and progression. Non-responding DME should have UWFA, and may benefit from PRP in presence of significant ischaemia.

OCT-A – optical coherence tomography angiography (*non-invasive imaging technology, using motion contrast between moving erythrocytes in blood vessels, against static retina*), provides topographic and structural information about retinal vessels (localized to superficial capillary plexus [SCP], or deep capillary plexus [DCP], and choriocapillaris or deep choroidal vessels).

■ Identifies neovascularization (IRMA, NVD, NVE), DME, assesses macular perfusion, and can be used to monitor treatment response (regression of NV).

■ **Widefield OCT-A** showing reduced macular and peripheral capillary density is predictive of severity and progression of DR.

■ Choroidal circulation shows reduced thickness and vascular density and flow voids in the choriocapillaris in ischaemic vasculopathy.

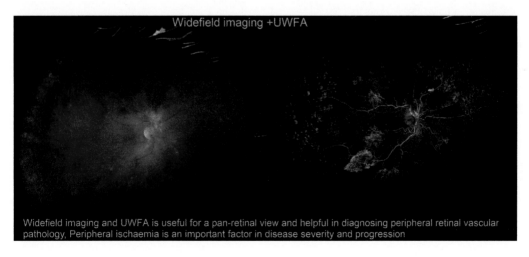

Figure 4.15 Widefield imaging and UWFA.

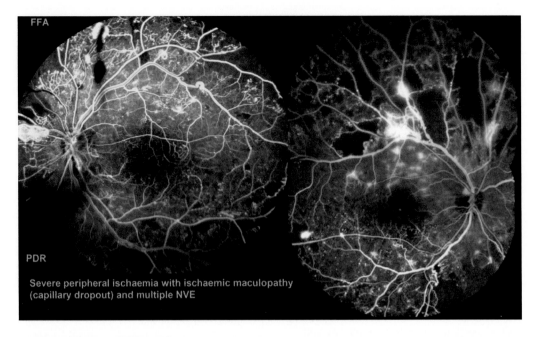

Figure 4.16 FFA in PRP – 2.

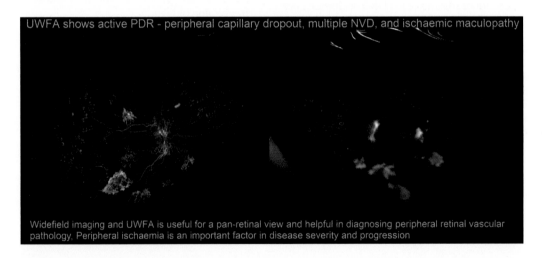

Figure 4.17 UWFA – PDR.

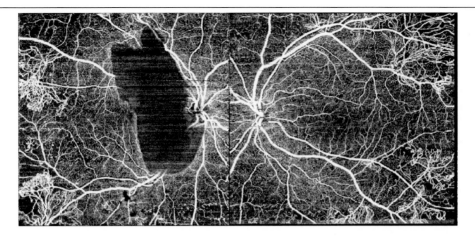

Figure 4.18 PDR-OCT-A.

OCT-A shows large preretinal haemorrhage at disc with multiple NVE in BE.

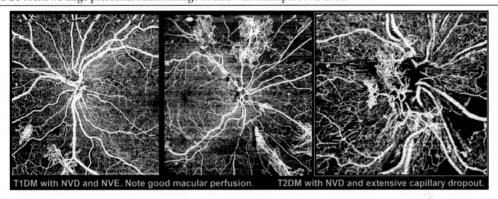

T1DM with NVD and NVE. Note good macular perfusion.   T2DM with NVD and extensive capillary dropout.

Figure 4.19 OCT-A with NVD and NVE.

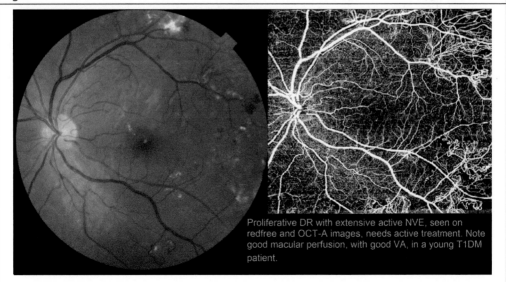

Proliferative DR with extensive active NVE, seen on redfree and OCT-A images, needs active treatment. Note good macular perfusion, with good VA, in a young T1DM patient.

Figure 4.20 PDR with NVE on OCT-A.

4.3.6 Understanding Laser Parameters for PRP

Spot size (50–400 µm)
• **The preferred spot for PRP is 200 µm.** The new concept favours the use of small spots, with gaps to preserve visual function.
• Large spots means energy is spread over a larger area, reducing laser intensity. A higher power is therefore required, to achieve the same effect, causing more painful treatment and larger areas of scarring. • **Large spots are more photo-destructive, painful, and best avoided.** • **Spots smaller than 200 µm are not advisable or safe**. A small spot is a more energized beam, and can cause deep retinal burns and a break in Bruch's membrane with a risk of CNV. • Additionally, treatment using small spots takes longer, with increased risk of phototoxicity.
• PASCAL offers multi-spot patterns to cover large retinal areas quickly, reducing the need for larger spots.
• **Spot size in relation to contact lenses used.** • Contact lenses used during treatment affect the size of burns delivered on the retina. • **Do not use spot >200 µm, with any wide-field lenses. They double the size of the spot delivered, require higher energy, and cause larger scars.**

Spacing between spots (0–2)
• **Spacing is important to preserve field of vision.** • Small spacing causes confluent burns that enlarge with time causing large scotomas and visual field loss. A **gap less than 1 spot size is not advisable.** • Wider spacing offers no advantage but makes subsequent fill-in PRP tedious and difficult. **A gap of more than 1.5 spot size is not ideal.**
• **Ideal spacing is 1–1.5 spot gap between burns, in young patients who need to drive.**

Pulse duration (10–1000 ms)
• A long pulse means that the retina is exposed to the laser for longer, with more heat dissipation. The argon laser has a long pulse of 50–200 ms, making it more destructive.
• **The default pulse duration with PASCAL is 20 ms (range used 20–30 ms), which is fine for most PRP treatments.**
• **A longer pulse causes painful treatment, deep burns, and risk of laser related hazard.**
• **A longer pulse (25–30 ms) may be used, with poor laser uptake**, in the presence of a pale or oedematous retina (CRVO), vitreous haemorrhage, or media opacities.

Grid Selection (with PASCAL Laser)
• PASCAL offers a selection of pre-determined **grid patterns for quick coverage of large areas of retina**, allowing faster, less painful treatment with fewer sessions.
• A variety of PRP grid patterns – square, hexagon, arc, and triangle – are available. There is no real advantage of one over another, and **most users select a square grid.** • **The number of spots in a grid ranges from single shot to large grids of 25 spots.**
• **Larger grids offer no major benefits, are more painful, slower to deliver, and more difficult to focus, especially in the periphery** (leading to uneven delivery of the grid).
For practical purposes, PRP treatment is done with: • **3 × 3 square grid – for treating mid and far peripheral retina.** • **2 × 2 square grid – for treatment at posterior pole (near periphery).** • **Single shots for fill-in PRP.**

Power Selection (0–2000 mw)
• It is difficult to assign a standard power setting, as response is dependent on multiple variables, like media clarity, fundus pigmentation, laser parameters, and delivery. **The power needed may vary in different retinal areas due to variability in reaction.** • **Power for PRP treatment is selected after titration (starting at 250 mw), until the desired reaction is seen, to a maximum of 500 mw.** If the spot is reduced at any stage – reduce the power.
• **Threshold power is the least power that causes a light white burn.**

Higher power is needed with:
- **Media opacities** – corneal oedema/scar, cataract, vitreous haemorrhage/opacities.
- **Pale retina** – reduced chorioretinal pigmentation leads to reduced laser uptake.
- **Oedematous retina** – in RVO or severe diabetic retinopathy.
- Media opacities dissipate laser energy, resulting in lower energy reaching the retina, and laser uptake is poor with pale, oedematous retina. These patients tolerate higher energy without complaining of pain.
- **Do not exceed powers greater than 500mw, especially if you are inexperienced with laser techniques, or patient complains of pain. Stop treatment and seek help.**

Lower power should be used with:
- **Pseudophakic and aphakic patients** – clear media, IOL focuses laser beams, causing a more intense reaction.
- **Pigmented fundi** – greater uptake (be careful with Asian and Afro-Caribbean patients).

- **Avoid excessive power that causes intense white burns as it can cause pain, induce vitreous haemorrhage, and become a focus for retinal breaks or CNV.**

PRP Treatment Plan

Number of shots per session.
- **A good session comprises 1000–1500 burns.** *(Exceptions to this are discussed later)*.
- **Number of treatment sessions required depends on disease activity.**
- **Do not undertreat** – you will not achieve much by doing 400–500 burns (except with fill-in PRP, with previous extensive treatment).

- The treatment plan is based on the patient's age and severity of disease.
- **Young patients tend to have more severe disease and need aggressive PRP.**
- **Each session comprises approximately 1000–1500 burns.**
- **Prophylactic PRP (PPDR)** – 2 sessions (2000–3000 burns).
- **Early PDR** – 2–3 sessions (3000–4500 burns).
- **Severe PDR** – 4–5 sessions (4000–6000 burns)
- **Review in 2 months after completion of treatment plan. Top up if it still looks active.**

- **End point of PRP is to regress new vessels, prevent vitreous haemorrhage, and stabilize the retinopathy. Treatment needs to continue until this goal is achieved.**

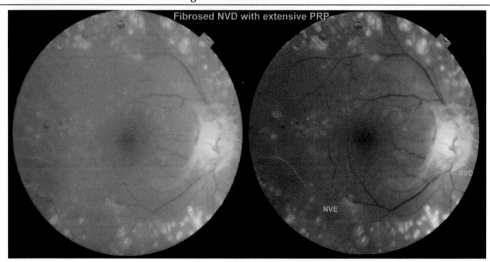

Figure 4.21 Fibrosed NVD.

- NV do not regress immediately after treatment. Fibrosis can take a few weeks to develop. It is important to give laser treatment time to work.
- **Unnecessary treatment should be avoided.** Consider **top up treatment**, only if NV look active in 2 months after initial treatment plan. *Do not simply laser because there is space on the retina. Treatment is always linked to disease activity.*

4.3.7 Exceptions to Treatment Plan

Fractionated laser (conservative treatment) with aggressive PDR
- Aggressive PRP in patients with high-risk PDR (extensive, forward-growing NVD/NVE) will induce excessive fibrosis causing traction, ERM, macular pucker, tractional macular hole, and tractional retinal detachment. These are sub-optimal outcomes, causing visual loss and requiring further treatments, with associated co-morbidity.

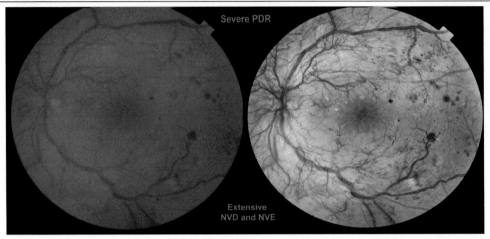

Figure 4.22 Severe PDR-1.

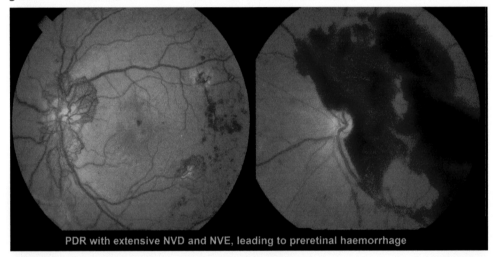

Figure 4.23 PDR with NVD, NVE, and preretinal haemorrhage − 1.

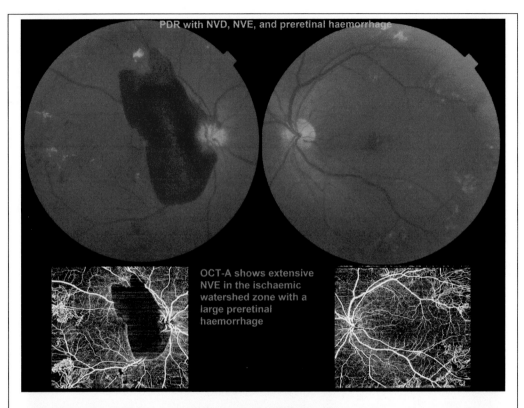

Figure 4.24 PDR with NVD, NVE, and preretinal haemorrhage – 2.

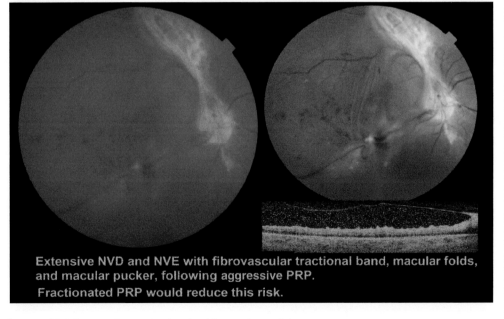

Figure 4.25 Fibrovascular traction bands with macular pucker.

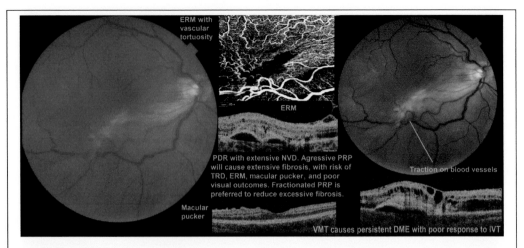

Figure 4.26 PDR with preretinal fibrosis.

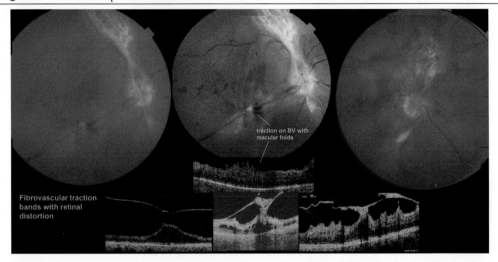

Figure 4.27 Fibrovascular traction bands.

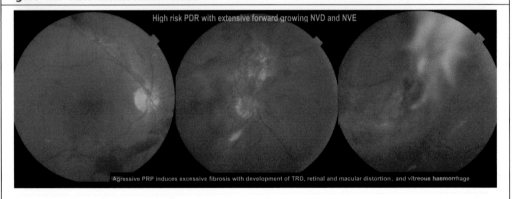

Figure 4.28 High risk PDR with NVD and NVE.

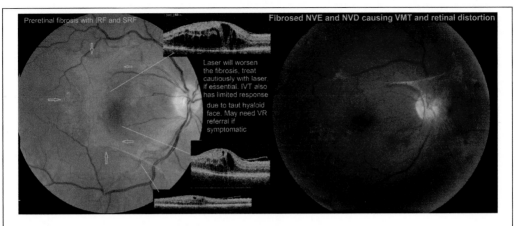

Figure 4.29 Fibrosed NVD and NVE with retinal distortion.

- It is advisable to avoid excessive, heavy laser to prevent these problems.
- Avoid >1000 burns in 1 session or completing PRP within 2–3 sessions.

The treatment plan remains the same, with patients requiring 4500–6000 burns, but delivery is done in a fractionated manner over multiple sessions at short intervals.

- Consider approximately 800–900 burns per session, spread over 5–6 sessions and completed over a period of 4–6 weeks.

4.3.8 Aggressive Laser Treatment in Ischaemic Retinal Vasculopathy

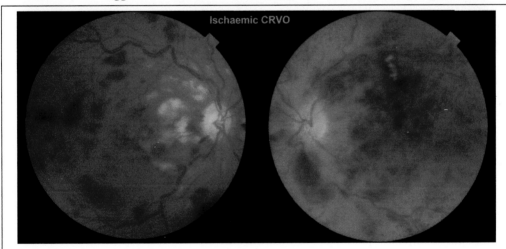

Figure 4.30 Ischaemic CRVO – 1.

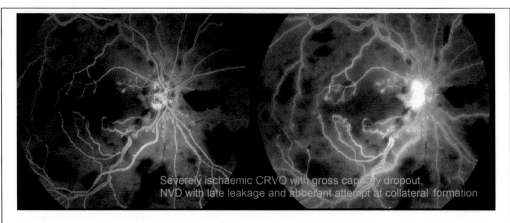

Figure 4.31 Severely ischaemic CRVO with NVD.

- Patients with ischaemic CRVO or ocular ischaemic syndrome have a high risk of retinal and anterior segment neovascularization (NVD, NVE, NVI, NVA) and neovascular glaucoma. They need a more aggressive approach in treatment.
- Delay in treatment results in development of rubeosis, and urgent laser treatment is needed to prevent this complication. **These patients need aggressive PRP in a short span of time.**

The preferred regimen is 2–3 sessions of 2500–3000 burns/session, to be completed within 1–2 weeks. The total treatment amounts to 5000–6000 burns.

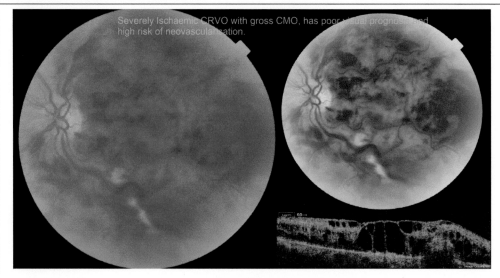

Figure 4.32 Severely ischaemic CRVO with high risk of NV.

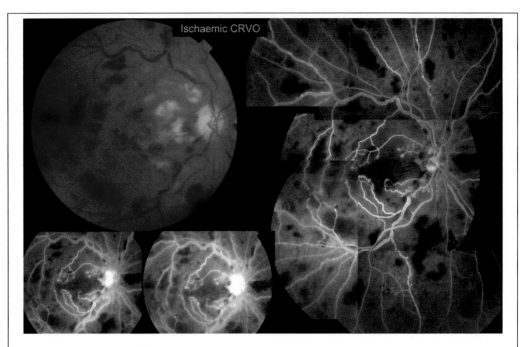

Figure 4.33 Ischaemic CRVO – 2.

The Chronic Non-attenders – Aggressive PRP

An additional category of patients who need aggressive PRP when seen in clinic are the young, active PDR patients who tend to be chronic non-attenders, likely to miss their appointments. They usually present back in clinic after a period of absence, with florid disease, complications of diabetic retinopathy (vitreous haemorrhage, TRD, rubeosis), severe visual loss, and a worse outcome from missed or delayed treatment.

- **It is vital to treat these patients aggressively, when seen in clinic, with maximum treatment (single PRP session) while the patient is with you.**
- **It may also be advisable to consider prophylactic PRP in high-risk patients (severe PPDR) if you are worried about their attendance.**

The long-term harm and costs involved justify an initial aggressive management approach.

4.3.9 Pan Retinal Photocoagulation – Procedure

Document vision and complete ocular examination to confirm pathology. **Review OCT-A or FFA images, if available, to plan treatment.**	

Informed consent is taken, explaining the risks and benefits of the procedure. **The aim is to stabilize diabetic retinopathy and vision. Improvement of vision is not the goal with current lasers.**	

Ensure BE are well dilated (tropicamide 1% + phenylepherine 2.5% ×2). A small pupil makes the procedure difficult. Diabetics do not dilate well due to associated neuropathy. Repeat drops or consider 10% PE if necessary (avoid in patients with cardiac problems).	

A treatment plan is essential to make appropriate lens and laser parameter selections. Decide on the treatment areas, number of shots, and number of sessions required.	

Select an appropriate contact lens, used with topical anaesthesia and coupling lubricant (based on treatment area, magnification required, and pupil size). **Mainster ×1 is ideal when starting PRP treatment.** Preferred CL for PRP:	

Mainster ×1	Good for mid-periphery and near periphery (posterior pole) – 30° to 130°. It offers a magnified view and is the **ideal lens when starting PRP**.
Goldmann 3-mirror lens	Offers better magnification than wide-field lenses, and the image is not affected by the patient's refractive errors. Use a tall mirror for far periphery (140–180°). Use a broad mirror for mid-periphery (90–140°).

Mainster-165 widefield lens	Good for complete PRP, without changing lenses, but the view is minified (fundal details and retinal burns may be difficult to see). Doubles spot size and needs higher power, so can be painful for patients. Not ideal for learners and inexperienced users.
QuadrAspheric lens	Good lens to use with small eyes, small palpebral apertures, and patients with poorly dilated pupils.

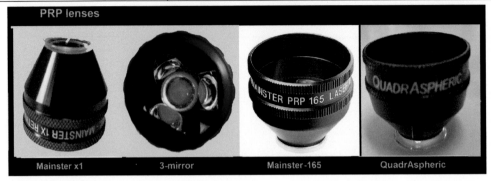

Figure 4.34 PRP lenses.

• Switch machine on, **select posterior treatment, and select pattern option. Machine autoselects 200 μm spot size and 20ms pulse duration.**
Slit Lamp Settings • Adjust table height, chinrest, IPD, eye-piece refractive error, to ensure sharp focus. • Keep slit at full height, medium width, and moderate illumination. • Slit lamp magnification ×6 to ensure a **wide FOV, keeping disc and macula in reference.**
Laser Parameter • Set aiming beam at just visible level (avoid glare), and select square grid pattern. • **Spot size – 200 μm; pulse duration – 20 ms; spot space – 1 to 1.5×.** • **Select 3×3 grid for new patients (treatment-naïve eyes).** • **Select 2×2 grid for fill-in PRP, and treatment at posterior pole.** • **Ensure every spot in the grid is in sharp focus.** • **Press ready when both doctor and patient ready.** • **Adjust power by titration** or guided by previous treatments to obtain a light white burn.

4.3.10 Starting PRP Treatment – Lesson Based on Treatment-Naïve Eye

When you first start PRP treatment, it is sensible to follow a schematic treatment pattern to make the procedure easy and controlled. If you are inexperienced with PRP, start with a 2×2 grid. This can be increased to 3×3 once you become comfortable.

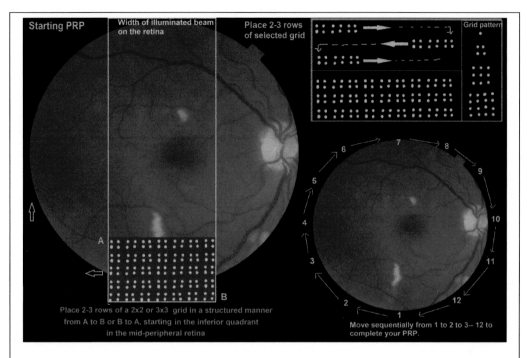

Figure 4.35 Starting PRP.

- Select the appropriate laser parameters as discussed above.
- **Start with the Mainster ×1 lens – magnified view of mid-periphery.**
- **Start treatment at the inferior mid-periphery.**

- Start at one end of the illuminated retina and move horizontally, placing the grid pattern in a row, to reach the other end of the illuminated area. Turn the joystick clockwise or anticlockwise to double back on yourself, and repeat the process, making a second row of laser burns. You can start peripherally and move in, or vice versa (A to B or B to A).
- **Place three to four rows of the selected grid in a defined and controlled manner.**
- Once the selected area is treated, move to the adjacent area and repeat the process.

- **Follow a logical sequence of retinal coverage, moving clockwise,** by asking the patient to move their eye (I–IN–N–SN–S–ST–T–IT). By doing so, a reasonable number of shots can be done quickly, with minimum lens movement on the eye.

- **When starting PRP, put 3–4 rows in the superior and inferior quadrant and 1–2 rows in the nasal and temporal quadrants. This is important to preserve driving visual field.** On completion of planned treatment, CL is removed and the follow-up plan activated.

- **Treating far periphery** – use three-mirror or wide-angled lenses (Mainster-165, QuadrAspheric, panfundoscope). Use a 2×2 grid (larger grids are harder to focus peripherally).

- **Treating near periphery** (posterior pole) – use a 2×2 grid with Mainster ×1 lens.
- For fill-in PRP use single shots or small grids.

- **A 3-mirror lens offers high magnification (better visualization of the retina and laser burns), but small FOV (in the mirror), requiring 360° rotation to cover the fundus**. With practice, this is an easy skill to acquire and a good technique for PRP and Retinopexy. **It does not affect the spot size, allowing use of lower laser power to complete treatment.**
- **Use a tall mirror for far periphery and a broad mirror for mid-periphery.**

- **Wide-angled lenses offer a panoramic, minified fundal view,** making subtle changes and laser burns difficult to see. They also require higher power to get the same effect (spots are doubled in size, reducing laser energy density).
- Spot doubling increases energy requirement by ×4.

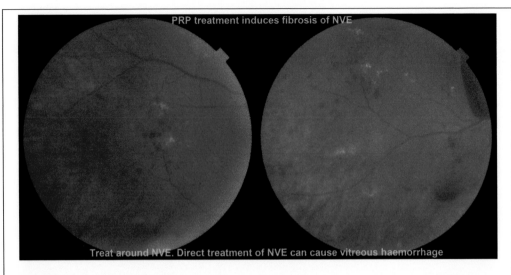

Figure 4.36 PRP with NVE fibrosis.

Good Practice with PRP
- **Mid-peripheral retina is most ischaemic and should be treated early.**
- **Early, active treatment is advised with severe NPDR, during pregnancy, prior to cataract surgery, and in patients with PDR in the other eye.**
- Avoid treating new vessels directly (risk of haemorrhage). Treat around them.
- Avoid re-treating previously lasered areas (more damaging and painful).

Patients with PDR and Coexistent Maculopathy

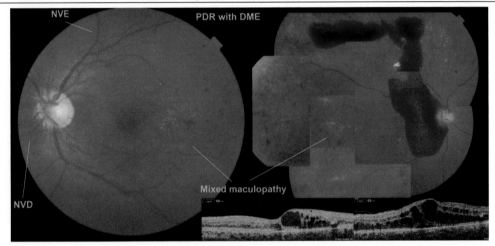

Figure 4.37 PDR with DME.

- PRP is known to exacerbate pre-existing DME, especially with aggressive PRP at short intervals (inflammatory pathway), although this usually improves with time (3/12).
- A 4–6-week interval between sessions reduces the risk and should be planned if possible.
- **Maculopathy should be treated a few weeks (4–6 weeks) prior to PRP if possible.**
- **If aggressive PRP is essential in high-risk cases, then IVT may prevent or stabilize DME during PRP.**

NVE Close to Macula
- **Needs cautious, fractionated treatment** (risk of macular traction, distortion, folds and pucker, ERM with VMT, lamellar, or FTMH).

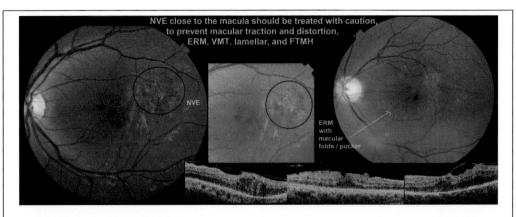

Figure 4.38 NVE close to macula

- **PRP with vitreous or preretinal haemorrhage should be treated with caution**, as blood absorbs green wavelength strongly. Await clearance of haemorrhage prior to PRP.
- Yellow (577 nm) or red wavelengths (810nm) are not absorbed by blood and may be used cautiously in the presence of some fundal view. **Do not treat if the fundal view is hazy due to a vitreous haemorrhage** (safe laser delivery not possible).

PRP in Patients with NVG
- PRP in patients with rubeotic glaucoma with corneal oedema can be difficult.
- Systemic diamox may reduce IOP and clear corneal oedema to allow safe PRP.
- Topical glycerine (glycerol 20% used 30 minutes prior to procedure) is another short-acting agent that may clear corneal oedema to improve retinal visualization.
- **If PRP is not feasible, and IOP remains high, consider treatment with cylclodiode laser.**

- **PRP in anxious, unco-operative patients** – slit lamp delivery can be difficult in anxious patients. These patients can have LIO in theatre under GA/sedation if required.

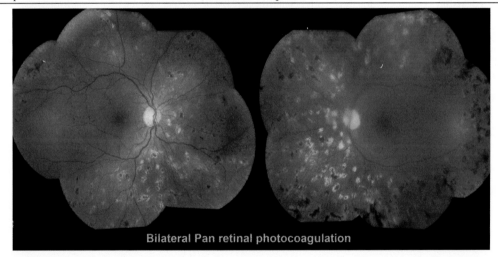

Figure 4.39 Bilateral PRP.

4.3.11 Risks of PRP

- **Floaters** – common after PRP due to vitreous syneresis or a diabetic bleed.

- **Vitreous haemorrhage** – PRP has a significant risk of inducing haemorrhage, by disturbing the vitreous, traction on NVD/ NVE, or inadvertent direct treatment of NVE, preretinal or subhyaloid haemorrhage. Aggressive PRP in patients with florid new vessels causes a fibrotic shift and traction, causing it to separate from the posterior hyaloid face, inducing a vitreous or subhyaloid bleed.

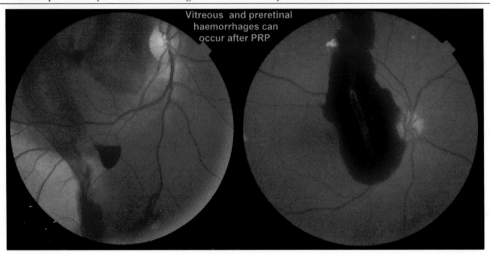

Figure 4.40 Vitreous and preretinal haemorrhage after PRP.

Effects on Visual Functions

Loss of vision – commonly due to vitreous haemorrhage (23%) or macular oedema (32%) (confirmed by OCT scan after PRP), inadvertent macular burn (acute loss), or late loss from laser scar extension. Other causes include excessive fibrosis causing ERM (9%), VMT, pucker, macular detachment, or macular hole, tractional retinal detachment (14%), and iatrogenic CNV (from heavy peri-macular laser burns), causing a sub-macular bleed.

- Visual outcomes are poor with co-existing macular ischaemia (7%) and neovascular glaucoma (5%), reflective of disease severity.

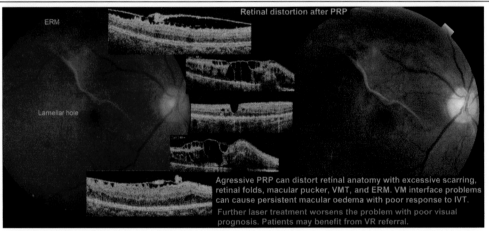

Figure 4.41 Retinal distortion after PRP.

Loss of Visual Field (fitness to drive) – 40–50% after full PRP, with large spots.

This can be reduced by using low power, small spots with ×1–1.5 gap between burns, and avoiding posterior pole treatment, if possible.

- **Other visual problems** – loss of contrast sensitivity, hemeralopia, nyctalopia, loss of colour vision in the blue spectrum, photophobia, and reduced ERG.

Worsening of macular oedema is common after aggressive PRP (25–43%). It causes transient visual disturbances, increased CRT on OCT, and drop in vision initially with improvement over several weeks. **Type of DME on OCT correlates better with visual outcome than the CRT.** Mechanism of DME following PRP is not entirely clear but likely to be due to vascular, inflammatory, and fibrotic changes (ERM with VMT) associated with PRP.

- **Dividing PRP treatment into 2 or more sessions at 3–4 weekly intervals and more peripheral PRP can minimize DME worsening.**

Tractional Retinal Detachment
- Aggressive PRP in patients with florid neovascularization induces excessive fibrotic shift and can cause TRD. These patients need gentler, fractionated PRP, with avoidance of large patterns, heavy burns, and excessive shots.

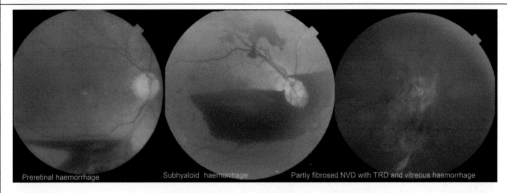

Figure 4.42 Preretinal, subhyaloid haemorrhage, TRD with vitreous haemorrhage.

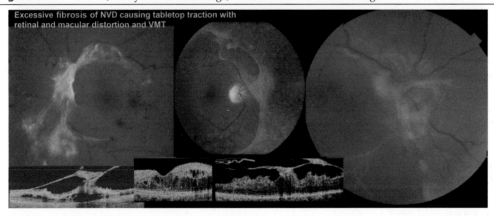

Figure 4.43 Excessive fibrosed NVD.

Pain during PRP is related to laser power, exposure time, and grid size.
- **Consider reducing these parameters (low power, short exposure, small grid), to make treatment comfortable. Avoid large grids in anxious patients with low pain threshold.**
- **Peripheral retina is thin and more sensitive**, previously treated areas with retinal thinning, PRP at 3 and 9 o'clock positions (site of long ciliary nerves), pseudophakes, and pigmented fundi have increased laser uptake, causing pain. Use low power in these patients.
- **Simple analgesics** (paracetamol) an hour prior to PRP treatment may relieve the pain.
- Rarely, **peribulbar or sub-tenon anaesthesia may be considered, or indirect PRP under general anaesthesia, in overly anxious patients.**

Iatrogenic choroidal neovascular membrane – can occur with deep laser burns in the peri-macular area causing a break in Bruch's membrane and sub-macular bleed.

Rare complications – corneal burns, raised IOP, angle closure glaucoma (associated with shallowing of AC, choroidal effusion, and myopia), CL-related problems (abrasions, infection). Extensive PRP can lead to RNFL loss, evident by disc pallor seen after PRP, and affect pupillary response, and poor dilation to mydriatics.
Progressive disease – 4–5% cases may continue to progress despite treatment, requiring medical (IVT) and surgical intervention with worse outcomes.

4.4 SECTORAL PRP

Patients with sectoral ischaemia, such as ischaemic branch retinal vein occlusion (BRVO) or hemiretinal vein occlusion (HRVO), only need treatment to the ischaemic quadrant. The laser parameters are the same as for PRP.

4.4.1 When Is Sectoral Laser Treatment Appropriate in BRVO?

Laser treatment is not indicated in the acute phase following a BRVO or HRVO. Patients must be assessed for presence of macular oedema and clinical signs of ischaemia – poor vision, multiple CWS, dark haemorrhages, gross CMO, and absence of collaterals.

Haemorrhages conceal the extent of ischaemia and absorb laser energy, making sectoral PRP unsafe in the acute phase. Collaterals develop and become evident as acute signs clear up in 2–3 months, and PRP may not be necessary. Sectoral PRP should be considered in 3 months if retinal ischaemia and CMO persist despite IVT.

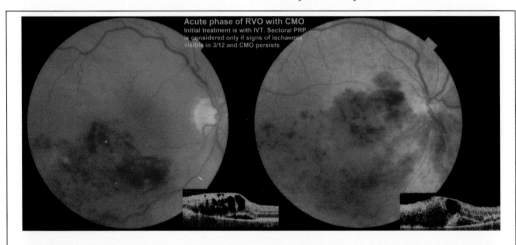

Figure 4.44 Acute phase of RVO.

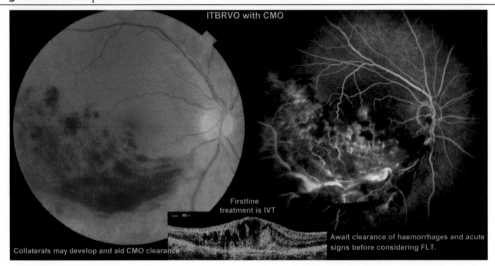

Figure 4.45 ITBRVO with CMO.

Generally, patients presenting with poor vision due to CMO are treated with IVT with anti-VEGF, or steroid implants in pseudophakic patients to aid clearance of macular oedema, improve vision, reduce the angiogenic drive, and help establish collaterals. It is reasonable to consider initial treatment with three loading doses of anti-VEGF therapy, and reassess the eye in 3 months. If vision remains poor and collaterals have not developed, an FFA is done to assess the extent of ischaemia, and sectoral PRP is considered, in the presence of significant ischaemia.

Sectoral PRP is also appropriate (without FFA) with overt clinical signs of ischaemia, or development of retinal neovascularization (NVD or NVE). Unlike CRVO, anterior segment neovascularization is less common with BRVO.

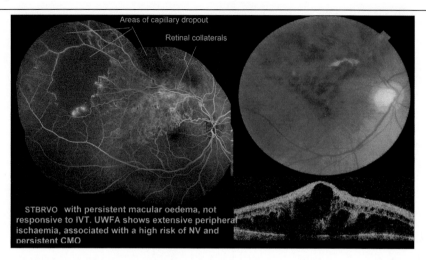

Figure 4.46 STBRVO with peripheral ischaemia.

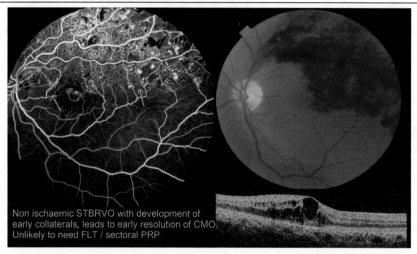

Figure 4.47 Nonischaemic STBRVO with good collaterals.

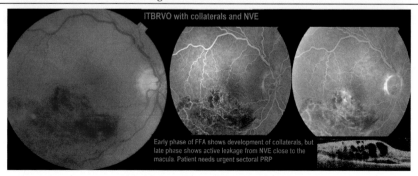

Figure 4.48 Inferotemporal BRVO with collaterals and NVE.

4.4.2 Sectoral PRP in BRVO or HRVO

- Look carefully for collaterals – visible clinically, more obvious on FFA.

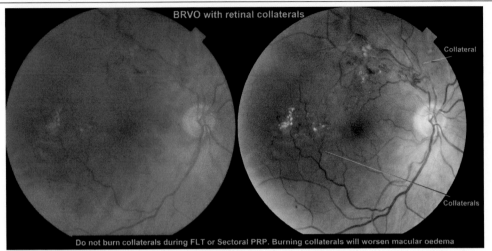

Figure 4.49 BRVO with collaterals.

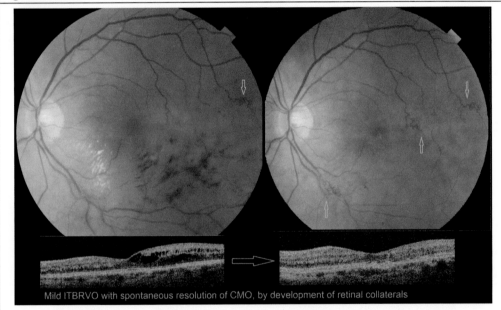

Figure 4.50 ITBRVO with resolution of CMO, following development of retinal collaterals.

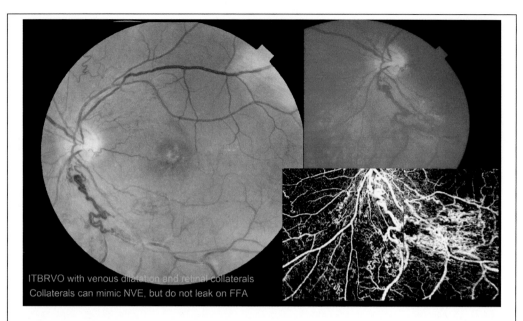

ITBRVO with venous dilatation and retinal collaterals
Collaterals can mimic NVE, but do not leak on FFA

Figure 4.51 ITBRVO with retinal collateral.

- **Collaterals are healing vessels, generally at the junction of perfused and non-perfused retina**. They help drain macular oedema and must be preserved during sectoral PRP. Burning collaterals worsens CMO, resulting in a worse visual prognosis.
- **If collaterals are not apparent clinically, look at the red-free or FFA images, which show the collaterals more clearly. In BRVO, they tend to be around the area of blockage.**

- **Target the ischaemic quadrant or hemifield. A single treatment session is adequate.**
- **BRVO – 800–1200 burns. HRVO – 1200–1500 burns.**

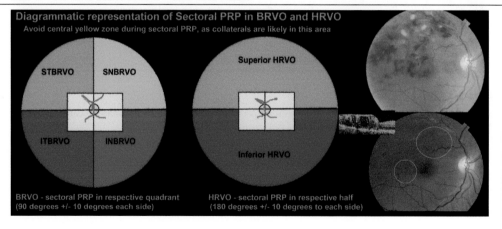

Diagrammatic representation of Sectoral PRP in BRVO and HRVO
Avoid central yellow zone during sectoral PRP, as collaterals are likely in this area

STBRVO SNBRVO
ITBRVO INBRVO

Superior HRVO
Inferior HRVO

BRVO - sectoral PRP in respective quadrant
(90 degrees +/- 10 degrees each side)

HRVO - sectoral PRP in respective half
(180 degrees +/- 10 degrees to each side)

Figure 4.52 Diagrammatic representation of sectoral PRP.

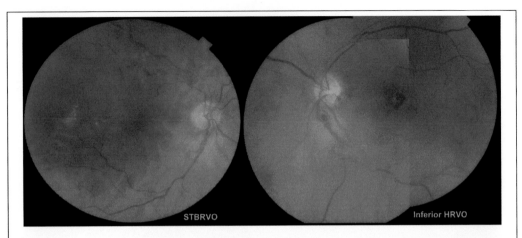

Figure 4.53 BRVO and HRVO.

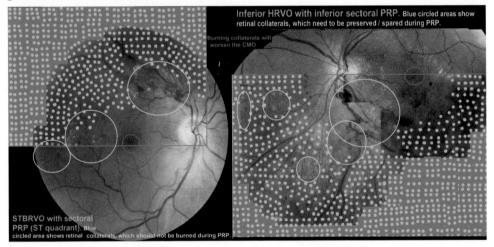

Figure 4.54 Sectoral PRP.

Laser parameters for sectoral PRP (treat mid and far periphery, avoid central yellow area – collaterals likely here). **Mainster ×1 or Mainster-165 lens used.**

- **BRVO – 800–1200 shots × 200 µm spot size × 20 ms duration × 250–350 mw power.**

- **HRVO – 1200–1600 shots × 200 µm spot size × 20 ms duration × 250–350 mw power.**

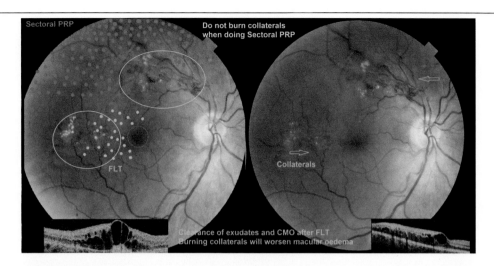

Figure 4.55 BRVO with sectoral PRP.

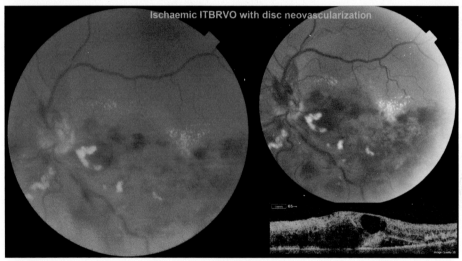

Figure 4.56 Ischaemic ITBRVO with NVD.

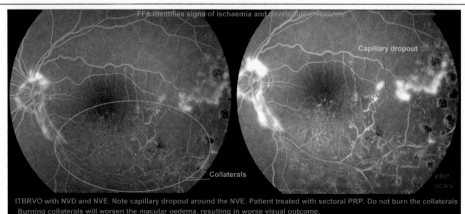

Figure 4.57 FFA in ITBRVO.

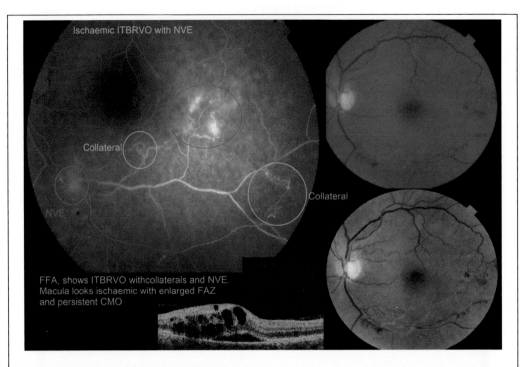

Figure 4.58 Ischaemic ITBRVO with NVE.

Collaterals and neovascularization may coexist in an ischaemic BRVO or HRVO. In the presence of severe sectoral ischaemia, the sectoral PRP can be extended a clock-hour on each side of the quadrant.

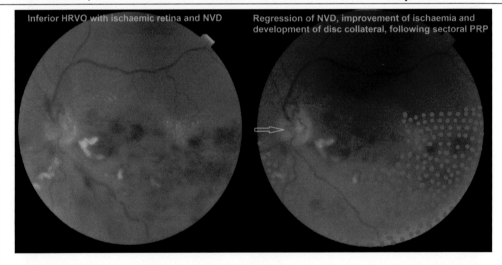

Figure 4.59 HRVO with NVD regression after Sectoral PRP.

4.5 FOCAL LASER TREATMENT

Previously, FLT was the gold standard treatment for diabetic maculopathy, but it has taken a back seat since the advent of anti-VEGF therapy, which is more efficacious for CiDME (centre involving DME). Laser remains the preferred treatment for NCiDME (non-centre involving DME), reducing the risk of visual loss by 50%. It can also be used in CiDME in conjunction with

IVT, or if IVT is declined or contraindicated. With the advent of multi-spot, sub-threshold, micro, and nano-pulse laser technologies, which are vision sparing and aid retinal rejuvenation, laser therapy is regaining importance.

FLT uses 532nm (green) or 577nm (yellow) wavelengths on melanin in the RPE (main site of action) and haemoglobin in the microaneurysms.

How does focal laser treatment work?

- The mechanisms of action are unclear but likely to be multifactorial.

- **Direct laser to microaneurysms** – reduces leakage by cauterizing and closing them.

- **Stimulates adjacent RPE to absorb SRF.**

- **Reduced oxygen demand and increased oxygen availability** – laser damage to photoreceptors reduces focal hypoxia, increasing oxygen availability to inner retina, and reversing formation of vasogenic oedema (Starling's law).

- **Down regulation of VEGF/inflammatory angiogenic factors and up regulation of several cellular or inter-cellular factors, with sustained neuroprotective effects after laser** – this theory is important, as it suggests the possibility of nondamaging, subthreshold laser treatment that promotes retinal rejuvenation.

4.5.1 Indications for Focal Laser Treatment

- Diabetic maculopathy.

  - Non-centre involving exudative maculopathy.

  - Centre-involving DME with CRT <400µm (not approved for IVT).

  - DME with CRT >400µm, patient reluctant/unsuitable for IVT.

- BRVO with CMO – patient reluctant or unsuitable for IVT.

- Macro-aneurysm.

- Persistent/recurrent CSR with parafoveal hot spot.

- Idiopathic juxtafoveal telangiectasia.

- Extrafoveal / parafoveal CNV (rarely).

4.5.2 Is It Essential to Target Microaneurysms?

Targeting microaneurysms is preferable, but not essential with current lasers.

FLT stimulates RPE and activates anti-angiogenic, immunogenic, and neuroprotective pathways that help clear the maculopathy. This forms the principle of treatment with grid laser in diffuse DMO, where laser is effective, despite mA not being visible.

Targeting microaneurysms will achieve the dual benefit of sealing them and the above effect.

- **Target mA if visible. If mA are not visible, a gentle modified grid is done, to cover the entire affected area.**

- **Newer lasers work by stimulating RPE and do not need specific targets. They work by high-density coverage of all ischaemic areas.**

4.5.3 Pre-Laser Investigations

The OCT scan has become central to decision-making in treatment of maculopathy.

- It documents and quantifies the maculopathy (measures central retinal thickness). **Central retinal thickness (CRT) is a better indicator of disease severity and outcome than vision alone.**

- Helps select appropriate treatment, based on OCT parameters of maculopathy.

- Compares 'before and after' images to judge the effectiveness of treatment.

- Identifies other macular or retinal changes, which may affect prognosis.

- OCT documentation allows monitoring of disease trend to help decide if a switch in treatment is necessary.

CRT is an important assessment tool to decide what treatment is appropriate.

If CRT is >400 µm – preferred treatment is intravitreal anti-VEGF agent.
If CRT is <400 µm – FLT is the preferred treatment.
Laser may be done with CRT >400µm, in patients reluctant to have IVT, medically unfit (cardiovascular problems, recent MI/CVA of less than 3/12 duration), unco-operative (needle phobia, confusion, dementia), or unable to commit to ongoing IVT due to lack of support.

4.5.3.1 Why Is It Important to Document other Macular Changes?

OCT documents structural macular changes that affect visual prognosis and laser outcomes – for example, ERM, FTMH, lamellar macular hole, macular pucker, preretinal or subretinal fibrosis, and vitreoretinal traction.

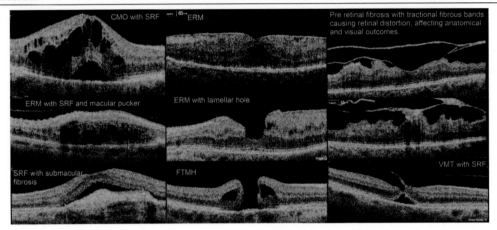

Figure 4.60 Why is it important to document other macular changes.

Awareness and documentation of pre-existing conditions are essential, as laser treatment can induce or worsen these changes. Macular oedema with co-existent structural changes has a worse anatomical and visual prognosis, and should be included in patient consent. Patients must understand that outcomes may be suboptimal, visual prognosis is guarded, and risk of vision worsening is a possibility.

The information helps appropriate selection of laser parameters, with small spots, low power and exposure time, and fewer shots, to reduce further scarring.

Patients may correlate adverse visual outcomes to their laser treatment. Documentation of pre-existing conditions and vision is essential to prevent any future misunderstanding and potential complaints or sources of litigation.

4.5.3.2 OCT Documents the Type of Macular Oedema

Prognosis and response to treatment varies with differing presentations of maculopathy. The topographic location of oedema on the retinal map, and morphological patterns of oedema on OCT, are useful predictors of treatment response in DME.

Presence of SRF and structural changes on OCT are associated with worse anatomical and visual outcomes.

Types of Macular Oedema	
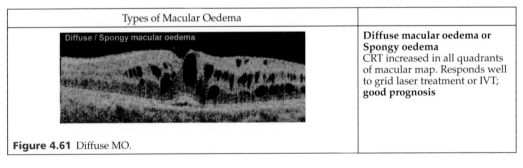 **Figure 4.61** Diffuse MO.	**Diffuse macular oedema or Spongy oedema** CRT increased in all quadrants of macular map. Responds well to grid laser treatment or IVT; **good prognosis**

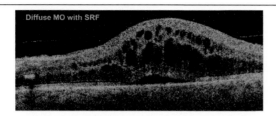 **Figure 4.62** Diffuse MO with SRF.	**Diffuse macular oedema with serous detachment (SRF)** **Presence of SRF is a worse prognostic indicator in DME.** The SRF acts as a barrier, hampering oxygenation of photoreceptors.
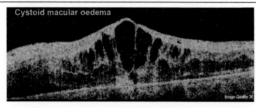 **Figure 4.63** CMO.	**Cystoid macular oedema (CMO)** Early CMO usually responds well to both grid laser and IVT. The response, however, is less effective than diffuse macular oedema.
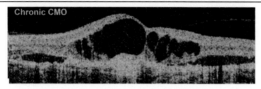 **Figure 4.64** Chronic CMO.	**Chronic CMO** Structural changes, with long-standing CMO, have a worse visual and anatomical prognosis to either laser or IVT. **May be associated with inflammatory response, which may benefit from IVTA or steroid implant.**
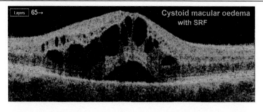 **Figure 4.65** CMO with SRF.	**Cystoid macular oedema with SRF** Prognosis is worse than diffuse oedema or CMO. **IVT is better than laser treatment.**
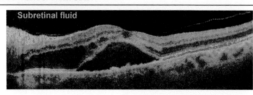 **Figure 4.66** SRF.	**Serous detachment (SRF) at macula (reflective of more severe disease)** **Presence of SRF is a worse prognostic indicator** (fluid acts as a barrier for inner retinal oxygenation).
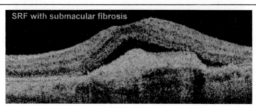 **Figure 4.67** SRF with sub-macular fibrosis.	**SRF with sub-macular fibrosis** Worse prognosis due to SRF and scarring. Laser will worsen fibrosis. **IVT is preferred treatment.**

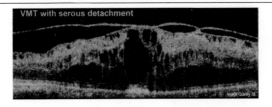

Vitreomacular traction with serous detachment
Worse prognosis, laser will worsen condition by inducing more fibrosis.

Figure 4.68 VMT with serous detachment.

Structural Macular Changes
- These are associated with poor visual and anatomical outcomes. Laser treatment likely to worsen VMT and ERM. If laser is done – use gentle, minimal treatment.
- IVT is preferred treatment, but prognosis is guarded whatever the treatment.

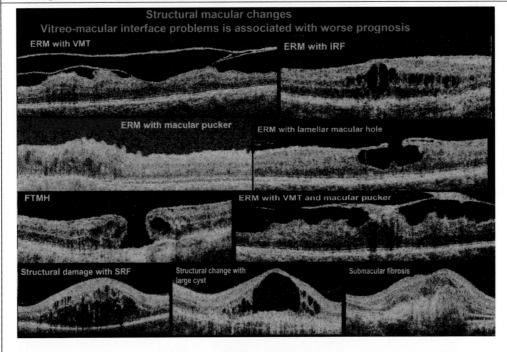

Figure 4.69 Structural macular changes on OCT.

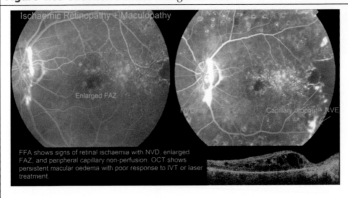

Figure 4.70 Ischaemic maculopathy + retinopathy.

Ischaemic Maculopathy

Featureless macula with poor vision and other signs of ischaemia – dark haemorrhages, CWS, IRMA, NV.

- FFA and OCT-A shows enlarged FAZ.
- Chronic DME, poor response despite multiple FLT.
- Poor prognosis.

OCT biomarkers include CRT, SRF, VRT, presence of hyperreflective foci, disruption of external limiting membrane, and choroidal thinning indicating worsening of DR and DME.

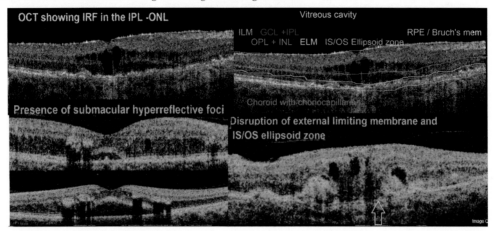

Figure 4.71 OCT analysis and biomarkers.

Hyperreflective foci indicate breakdown of blood-retinal barrier, causing lipoprotein extravasation, development of hard exudates, and a worse visual prognosis.

OCT-A – assesses macular perfusion, size, and morphology of FAZ (loss of capillary density in superficial and deep capillary plexus with enlarged FAZ), correlates number of mA in the DCP to DME, and documents other perimacular changes like NVE, collaterals, RAM. OCT-A changes may be visible long before classic signs of DR become manifest.

It allows objective assessment and quantification and is a good predictor of severity and progression of DME, DR, and response to IVT. Eyes with more mA in the DCP plexus and larger FAZ have a poorer response to IVT. Reduced macular and peripapillary capillary perfusion density (SCP > DCP) on OCT-A can diagnose macular ischaemia and glaucoma prior to RNFL thickness changes or visual field loss, in patients with high IOP.

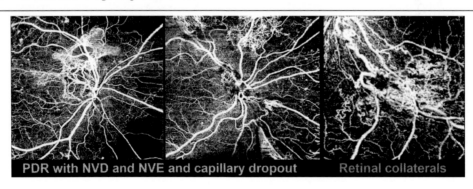

Figure 4.72 OCT-A.

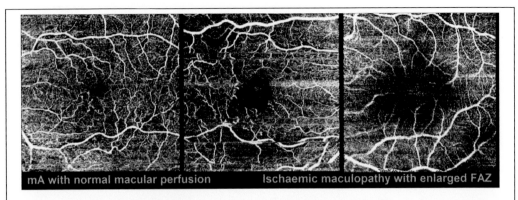

Figure 4.73 OCT-A macular perfusion.

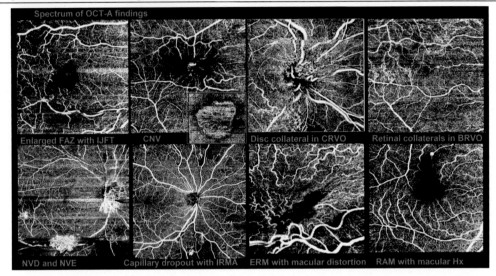

Figure 4.74 Spectrum of OCT-A findings.

4.5.3.3 Fundus Fluorescein Angiography

FFA is not essential for FLT but may be useful to identify leaking microaneurysms, early neovascularization, old laser scars, and the extent and areas of retinal or macular ischaemia. UWFA identify the extent of peripheral non-perfusion, and the calculation of ischaemic index correlates strongly with severity and progression of DR and DME. DME unresponsive to IVT should have UWFA to assess and treat peripheral ischaemia.

FFA is especially useful in patients who have had multiple (more than three to four) FLT, to find the underlying reason for their persistent maculopathy.

An FFA may help identify the leaking areas to allow targeted treatment.

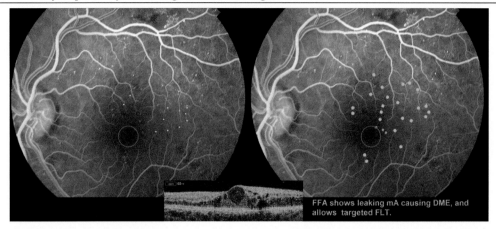

Figure 4.75 FFA shows leaking mA.

It may identify ischaemic maculopathy – where laser is less effective.

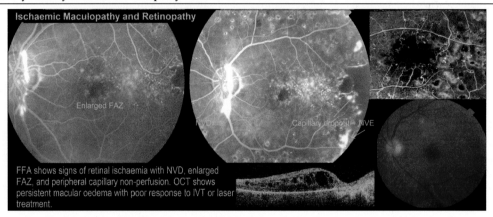

Figure 4.76 FFA shows ischaemic maculopathy.

It may identify perimacular NVE as the source of leakage.

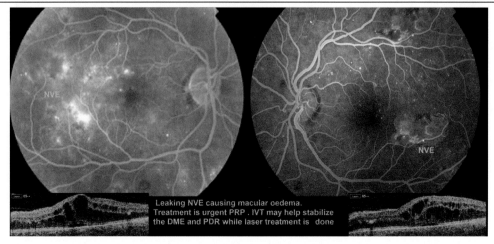

Figure 4.77 FFA shows leaking NVE.

4.5.3.4 Focal Laser Treatment in Diabetic Maculopathy

The **Early Treatment Diabetic Retinopathy Study** (ETDRS) defined CSME as:
- Retinal thickening at or within 500µm of centre of the macula.
- Hard exudates at or within 500µm of macula with adjacent retinal thickening.
- Retinal thickening >/= 1-disc diameter/within 1-disc diameter of the macula.

Circinate may be single or multiple and need treatment if vision is threatened. Exudates do not need direct treatment; sealing leaking microaneurysms helps exudates clear.

4.5.3.5 Starting Focal Laser Treatment

FLT stabilizes maculopathy and maintains vision. Early treatment (before foveal involvement) is most effective.

Significant visual improvement is unlikely and not the primary goal of FLT.

Examine patients to confirm the diagnosis and ensure the clinical picture has not altered, to avoid potential errors. Review OCT, FFA, if available and plan appropriate treatment.

An informed consent, stating risks and benefits of FLT, is essential.

Pre-laser drops – ensure BE are well dilated (tropicamide 1% + phenylepherine 2.5% ×2).

Slit lamp parameters – adjust:
- Table height, chinrest, eyepiece IPD, and refractive errors.
- Select full slit height and **medium slit width and just visible illumination**.
- Examine at low magnification (×6). **Select magnification of ×10 or ×16 for treatment.**

Laser Parameters
- **Set just visible aiming beam illumination. Select single spot.**
- **Machine pre-sets laser parameter – spot size 100um; pulse duration 10ms**
- **Use 50um for direct treatment of mA and treatment close to FAZ.**
- **Power – start with 100mw; titrate up until a light grey burn is visible.**

Use contact lens with topical anaesthesia and coupling lubricant.

Commonly used lenses are:

Mainster Focal and

Volk Area Centralis.

Both offer high magnification and a good view of the posterior pole.

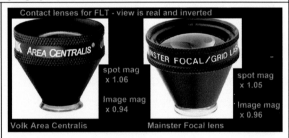

Figure 4.78 CL for FLT.

FLT can be safely applied to leaking microaneurysms between 500µm and 3000µm from the fovea, using a 100µm spot size.
Do not treat within 500µm of fovea. (For reference – retinal artery diameter at the disc is 150µm, so avoid 2 retinal artery-diameter distance all around the foveal pit.)

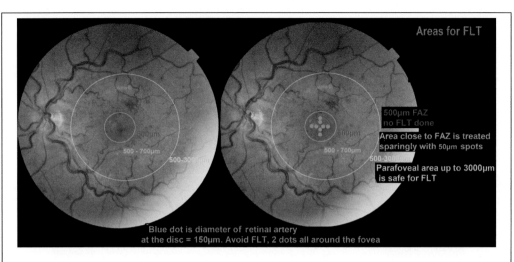

Figure 4.79 Areas for FLT.

- Titrate (trial shots), appropriate power away from the fovea (typically near the arcades). Most FLT can be done at 120–200 mw power.
- Target microaneurysms within circinate if visible – aim for blanching of mA or light grey burns. Avoid the central 500 um FAZ (Foveal Avascular Zone).
- Avoid over-treating, re-treating the same areas, and deep white burns.
- Start away from the fovea and gradually come in once you become comfortable.
- CRT can vary across the macula, requiring variable power. Adjust accordingly, to avoid deep burns. Use discrete (non-confluent) shots with a gap of ×1–1.5 spot.

Use lower power in	Use higher power with
• Pseudophakia (IOL focuses laser energy)	• Diffuse CSME (IRF/SRF)
• Aphakia (clear media)	• Pale fundus
• Pigmented fundi (Asian, Afro-Caribbean patients)	• Media opacity

Typical number of shots used. Excessive laser causes extensive scarring that can coalesce and involve the fovea. Try not to exceed the numbers shown below.
- FLT – 5–25 shots (depending on size and number of treatment areas).
- Modified grid – 15–35 shots.
- Grid laser – 35–75 shots.

Laser Parameters for FLT, using Mainster focal lens or Area centralis

FLT > 500 μm away from FAZ
- 5–25 shots × 10 ms (exposure time) × 100 μm (spot size) × 150 – 225 mw (power)

FLT close to FAZ – 2–5 shots × 50 μm × 10 ms × 100–150 mw (just to mA) (*Treat cautiously and sparingly using 60um spot size, target individual mA only.* **Small spot size – reduce power.**)

Grid laser – 25–75 shots × 10 ms × 100 μm × 150–225 mw

- Rarely, with poor laser uptake (excessive CSME, media opacity) – power may be increased to 250 mw or exposure time increased to 15ms.

- **Always use single shots** – this is the safest and most controlled way to do FLT.
- **Pre-selected grids close to the macula carry a higher risk of macular burns** with nervous patients, or inexperienced doctor.
- **You are less in control** and a wrongly placed pattern, or patient movement during laser delivery, can be devastating for visual outcome. A single misplaced laser burn is less damaging than multiple burns close to the fovea (*pre-selected grids are used with EPM*).

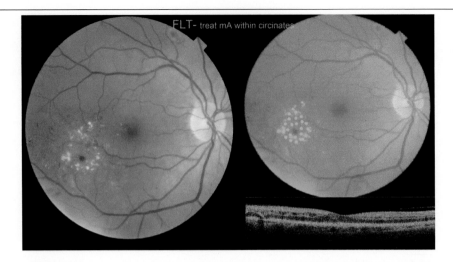

Figure 4.80 FLT – 2.

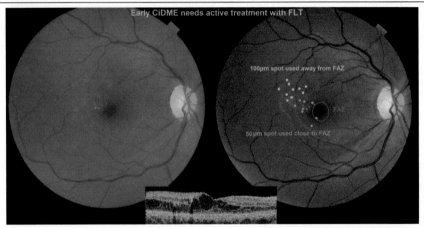

Figure 4.81 Early CiDME.

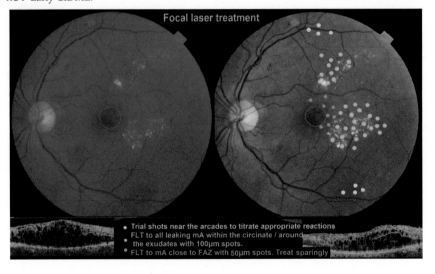

Figure 4.82 Focal laser treatment.

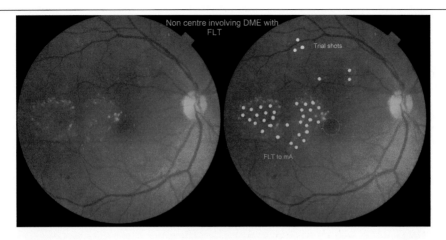

Figure 4.83 FLT to NCiDME.

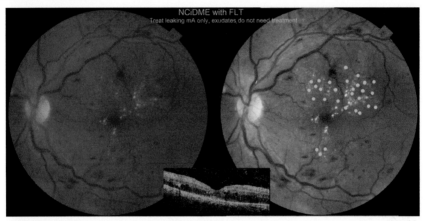

Figure 4.84 FLT for NCiDME.

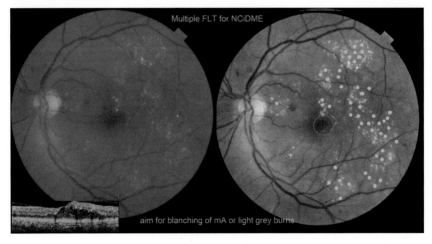

Figure 4.85 Multiple circinates treated with FLT.

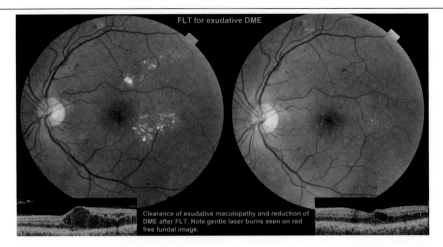

Figure 4.86 F LT for exudative maculopathy.

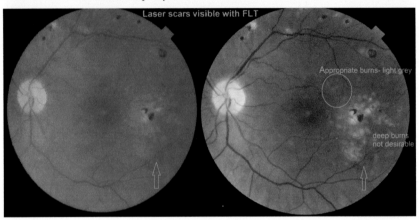

Figure 4.87 FLT laser burns.

Exudates can take up to 4–6 months to absorb and clear. FLT should not be repeated within 4 months of initial treatment. New areas of exudation can be treated with FLT. Avoid re-treating areas with previous laser scars.

4.5.3.6 Grid Laser Treatment

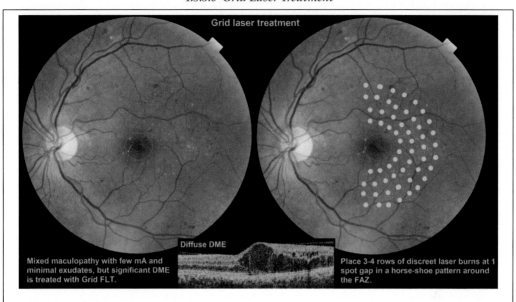

Figure 4.88 Grid laser treatment.

Traditional grid laser is done for diffuse DME, without obvious microaneurysms.
- A grid should not be repeated unless the initial treatment was suboptimal.
- 3–4 rows of single, discrete burns placed in a horseshoe-shaped pattern around the fovea, with a gap of one spot between burns.
- **Diffuse oedema may alter macular anatomy** (look at red-free images to identify FAZ).

Grid laser treatment – 35–55 shots × 100 μm spot size × 10 ms pulse duration × 100–200 mw power, with 1 spot size gap between barely visible burns × Mainster Focal lens

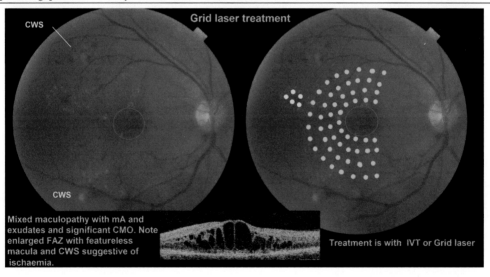

Figure 4.89 Grid laser treatment – 1.

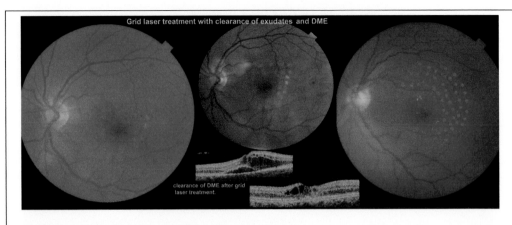

Figure 4.90 Grid laser scar with clearance of exudates.

4.5.3.7 *Extended Grid Laser Treatment*

In the presence of extensive CSME – extended grid laser treatment can be done, which can extend almost up to the arcades **(50–100 burns).** It can be classified as
- **Inner grid** – 3 rows around the fovea (yellow spots) – **25–50 burns**; and
- **Outer grid** – 3–4 rows outside the inner grid – **25–50 burns** up to the arcades (orange spots).

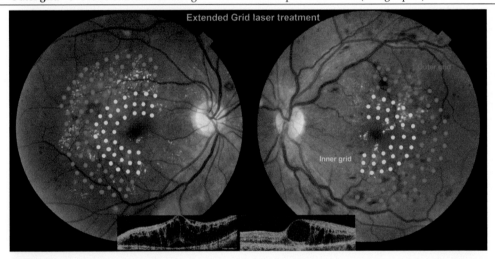

Figure 4.91 Extended grid laser treatment – 2.

An extended grid is generally not done these days, as these patients are more likely to be treated with IVT, but could be considered in patients who refuse or are unable to have IVT for medical, social, or economic reasons. Visual and anatomical prognosis is more guarded with diffuse CSME and more extensive laser treatment.

Extensive oedema distorts macular anatomy, making it difficult to locate the FAZ. If laser treatment is essential, a 2-stage treatment is preferable. Consider a gentle outer grid first to reduce CSME, then an inner grid at a later date (3 months) once the anatomy is restored.

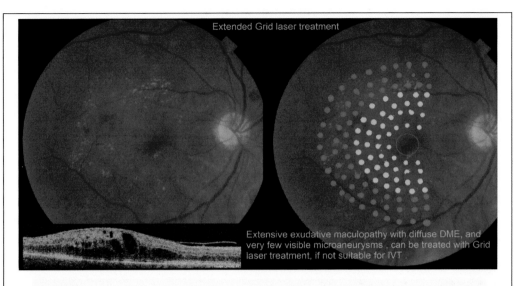

Figure 4.92 Extended grid laser treatment – 1.

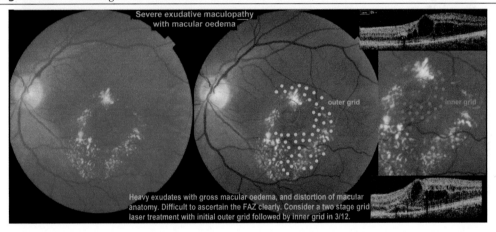

Figure 4.93 Severe exudative maculopathy with MO.

4.5.4 Grid Laser Treatment – Including the Papillo-Macular Bundle

- Retinal exudates or circinates, nasal to the fovea can be treated cautiously with a **grid laser in a circular pattern (all around the fovea).**
- **A heavy nasal grid is not advisable as it causes paracentral scotoma.**
- A traditional horseshoe grid spares the nasal area, which **contains the Papillo-Macular Bundle. Caution must be exercised when treating this area, using gentler treatment** (fewer shots, lower power, reduced exposure time).
- **Consider alternative treatment options (intravitreal steroid or anti-VEGF).**

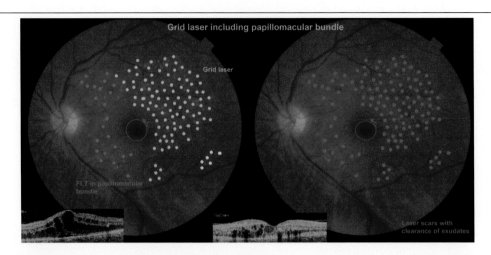

Figure 4.94 Grid laser including papillomacular bundle.

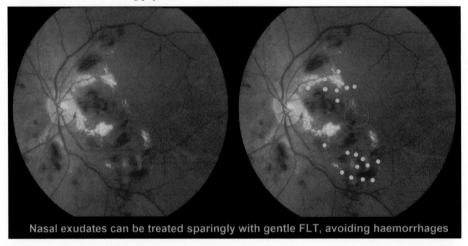

Figure 4.95 Nasal exudates treated with FLT.

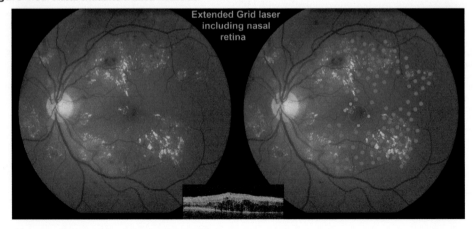

Figure 4.96 Extended grid including nasal retina.

Modified Grid Laser

- **Modified grid** is used for large parafoveal circinate, with multiple microaneurysms in the centre, or diffuse thickening with no obvious microaneurysms seen.
- **A pattern of gentle laser burns using threshold power, least number of shots, with one-spot gap is used to fill the entire thickened area within the circinate.**

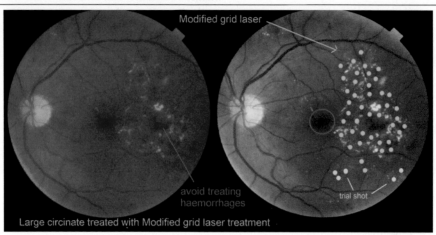

Figure 4.97 Modified grid laser.

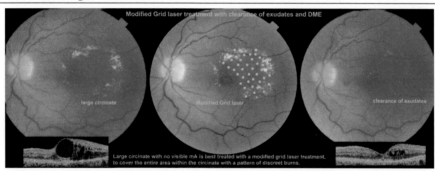

Figure 4.98 Modified grid laser with clearance of exudates.

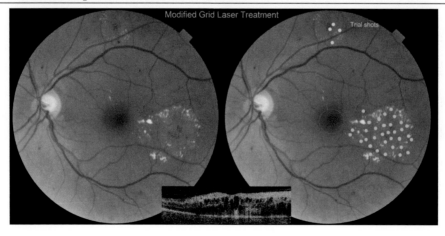

Figure 4.99 Modified grid laser-1.

4.5.4.1 Ischaemic Maculopathy

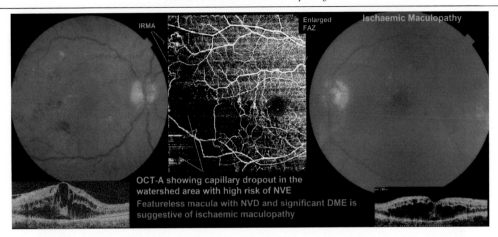

Figure 4.100 Ischaemic maculopathy-1.

Suspect ischaemic maculopathy if:
- Poor visual outcome, despite multiple FLT or IVT.
- Macular changes do not correlate to symptoms (symptoms worse than signs).
- Featureless, effaced macula, persistent CSME.
- Other fundal signs of ischaemia – CWS, dark haemorrhages at watershed zone, venous changes, IRMA, neovascularization.
- FFA or OCT-A will confirm enlargement of FAZ due to capillary dropout.

Patients with ischaemic maculopathy are unlikely to benefit from laser treatment, and repeated laser treatment may do more harm than good. Consider other treatment (IVT), and warn patients of guarded visual prognosis. Patients may need PRP as they are likely to also have generalized retinal ischaemia.

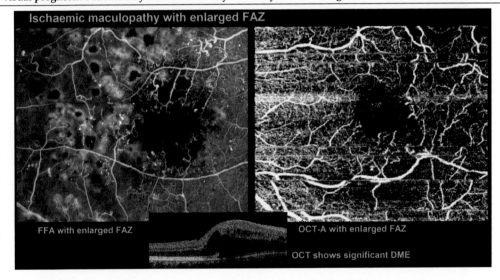

Figure 4.101 Ischaemic maculopathy – FFA and OCT-A.

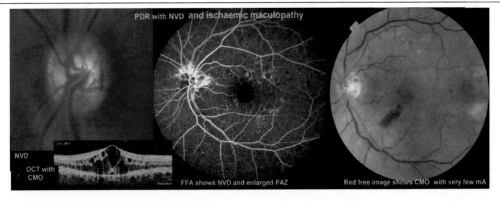

Figure 4.102 PDR with ischaemic maculopathy.

4.5.4.2 Focal/Grid Laser Treatment Using End Point Management (EPM)

EPM uses 532nm (green) or 577nm (yellow) laser light at subthreshold power, to selectively stimulate RPE. The laser burns are not visible clinically or by imaging modalities.

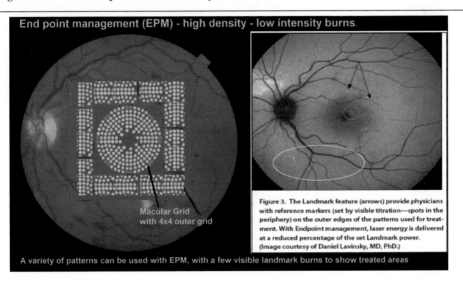

Figure 4.103 EPM FLT.

PASCAL EPM technique (if available)

- Select EPM option on PASCAL and pattern of multiple shots.
- Machine auto-selects 200μm spot, 15ms pulse duration, and spot spacing of 0–0.5.
- Titrate to get a barely visible burn = **Threshold energy** (100% energy)
- Select 30% of threshold energy. Non-damaging treatment (no CR scarring, scotoma (vision sparing)). **Avoid central 500μm of FAZ** (*diameter of central part of circular pattern*).
- As there are no visible burns, the pattern gives the option of a few peripheral visible burns that serve as markers for appropriate treatment delivery (**landmark pattern**).

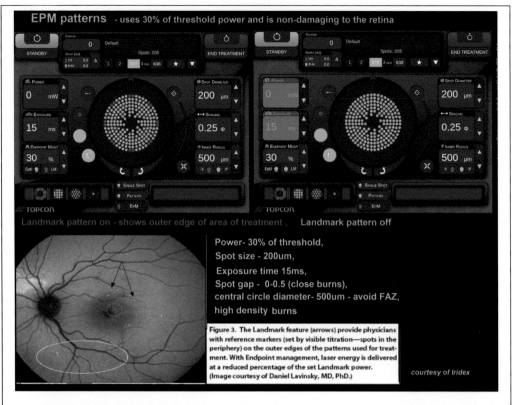

Figure **4.104** EPM menu page.

- **Subthreshold laser stimulates RPE without photothermal damage to overlying neuroretina, due to short pulse duration and low power.**

- Efficacy of EPM increases if more RPE cells are exposed to the thermal stress.
- **A high density, low intensity therapy, using larger grids, is more effective treatment. An average of 400-700 shots** are placed close to each other **as confluent burns or with a 0.25 spot distance.**

- Pattern technology allows equidistant spacing of spots for effective, faster macular grid, with less pain and preservation of macular function (colour vision and contrast sensitivity) and increased retinal sensitivity compared to conventional lasers.
- There are no known complications of EPM but **inappropriate titration with higher energy can cause thermal damage,** leading to visual loss. **EPM should not be applied over areas of haemorrhages or intense pigmentation that could cause deeper burns.**
- **EPM** can be repeated in 3 months.

4.5.4.3 Outcomes of FLT

Unlike in IVT, **effects of FLT are not immediate. They take 3–6 months,** with absorption and clearance of exudates and reduction of CSME.

- **FLT should not be repeated for 3–4 months from initial treatment. Excessive, multiple FLT will lead to extensive macular scarring and poor visual outcome.**

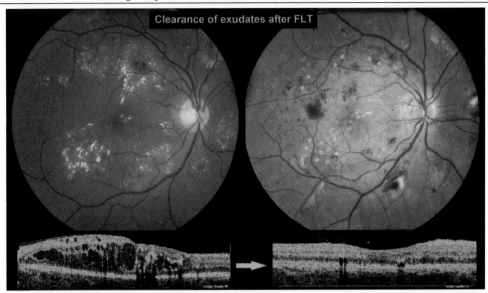

Figure 4.105 Clearance of exudates after FLT – 1.

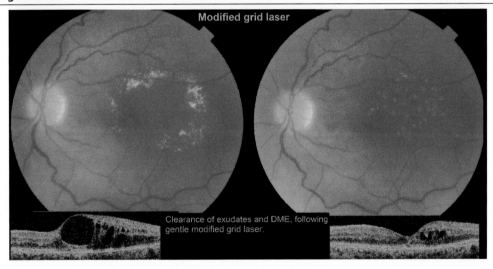

Figure 4.106 Clearance of exudates after FLT – 2.

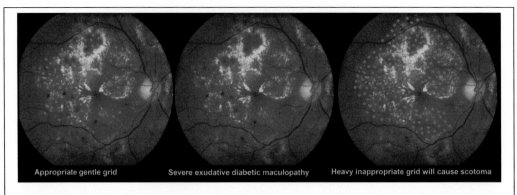

Figure 4.107 Extended grid Appropriate vs Heavy laser.

- **FLT can be repeated in 4–6 months, if involving a different part of the macula, or if initial treatment was sub-optimal (undertreatment).**
- More than 2 grid laser treatments are not advisable, and if DME persists investigation with FFA is essential, to offer targeted treatment or rule out macular ischaemia. Alternative treatment options (IVT) may be preferable in these patients.

- **A pre- and post-treatment OCT compares CRT to confirm anatomical improvement. However, visual outcome does not always co-relate to anatomical changes.**

- Poor diabetic control, uncontrolled hypertension, hyperlipidaemia, and smoking cause severe persistent exudative maculopathy. Advice regarding these conditions are helpful.
- FLT reduces CSME and CRT better than clearance of exudates. Persistent exudates may require treatment with statins and fibrates.

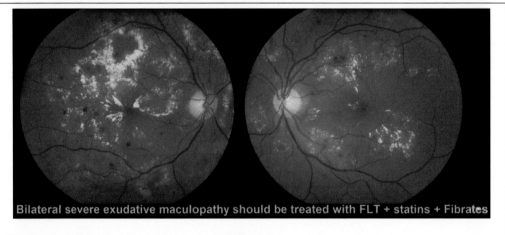

Figure 4.108 Bilateral severe exudative maculopathy.

Diffuse Maculopathy in Presence of Neovascularization

When maculopathy co-exists with disc or retinal neovascularization, what you treat first depends on the patient's age and severity of retinopathy.

- In **young patients** with active neovascularization, it is generally recommended to treat new vessels first, with PRP, as they advance rapidly with devastating consequences.
- In **older patients** it is better to treat the maculopathy first (4–6 weeks before), as PRP can hasten progression of maculopathy.
- **Fractionating PRP into sessions of 700–800 burns separated by 2–3 weeks and PRP in the far periphery reduces risk of DME progression.**
- **Consider intravitreal therapy (anti-VEGF or steroid) to treat maculopathy prior to starting an urgent PRP**. IVT stabilizes or resolves oedema, which is quicker than laser treatment and prevents PRP-associated worsening of DME.
- **Patients with significant PDR, are likely to have ischaemic maculopathy**. FLT needs to be applied cautiously, and visual prognosis is guarded. Consider an FFA and treatment with IVT may be preferable to laser.

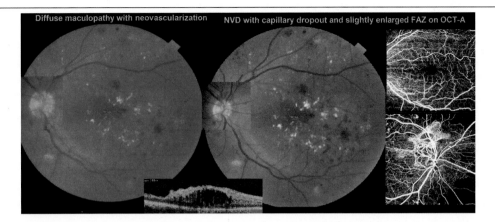

Figure 4.109 PDR with maculopathy.

Mixed Maculopathy (Exudative + Ischaemic)
- **First-line treatment is IVT, with guarded prognosis.**
- Once CRT has reduced, a gentle FLT can be considered for residual exudates. This approach avoids excessive laser treatment, which has a worse outcome in presence of severe oedema and ischaemia.
- The deferred FLT may help by reducing further leakage and the overall number of IVT injections required, to achieve long-term stability.

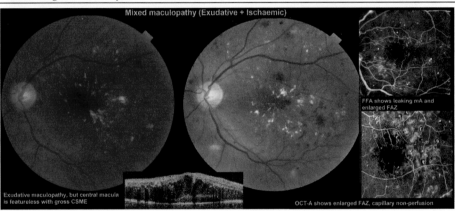

Figure 4.110 Mixed maculopathy.

Ischaemic Maculopathy
- Ischaemic maculopathy confirmed by FFA should not have further FLT.
- Consider IVT (anti-VEGF), which is less damaging. Patients are warned of a guarded prognosis, whatever the treatment. With extremely poor vision, consider stopping treatment and CVI registration.

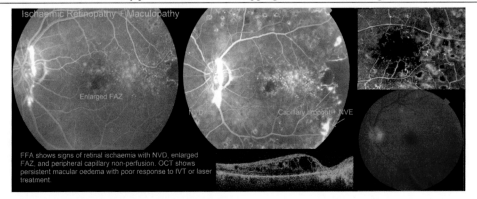

Figure 4.111 FFA shows ischaemic maculopathy.

Cataract with Maculopathy
- Patients with cataract and active DME, should have their maculopathy treated first, as **cataract surgery is known to worsen maculopathy (inflammatory pathway).**
- If laser treatment is difficult due to advanced cataract, affecting fundal view, then **preoperative or intraoperative steroid injection (IVTA) or anti-VEGF** can prevent worsening of DME in high-risk patients.
- Steroids are preferred in this scenario, as anti-VEGF does not address the post-surgical inflammatory component that drives the DME.

Patients need close monitoring in the post-surgical period, for IOP assessment, progression of maculopathy, or retinopathy, and may need laser treatment postoperatively.

Diffuse Non-Responsive Macular Oedema with ERM
- Patients with significant ERM with surface wrinkling, macular hole, macular pucker, or other VM interface problems with persistent SRF and significant visual loss or distortion should not have further FLT.
- Laser induces more scarring with worsening anatomical and visual outcomes.
- A vitreoretinal referral is advisable for a possible vitrectomy and ILM peel, which often will lead to the resolution of the persistent oedema.

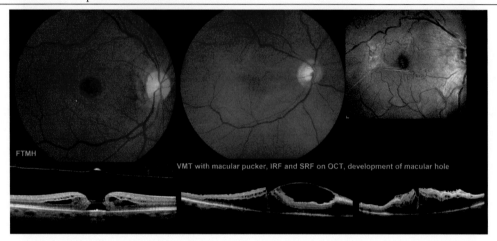

FTMH

VMT with macular pucker, IRF and SRF on OCT, development of macular hole

Figure 4.112 FTMH, Macular pucker.

FLT in Aphakia and Pseudophakia
- The principles of FLT remain the same, but care must be taken in pseudophakic DME patients. The IOL acts as a magnifying lens, concentrating laser energy, resulting in intense burns. Laser titration is important to reduce the power used.
- Aphakic patients also have more intense burns due to a clear media.
- These patients may have altered vitreoretinal interface, with the potential risk of tractional retinal detachment and macular holes (more with PRP), and cautious laser treatment is advisable.

Recent cataract surgery in diabetics with DME involves a large element of inflammatory oedema and these patients may benefit from IVTA or sub-tenon steroid injection in the immediate postoperative period. FLT is only considered if the DME persists 6–8 weeks after the steroid injection and an FFA confirms leaking microaneurysms.

Pregnancy and DME
- Pregnancy is a high-risk period for poor diabetic control and progression of diabetic eye disease, requiring close monitoring and proactive treatment.
- 10–25% T1DM patients develop DME during pregnancy. Treatment options for these patients are improved BSL, observation, and FLT for non-centre involving DME.
- For DME refractory to FLT, intravitreal steroids may be a safer option during pregnancy. Steroids are not recommended in first trimester, as they can be associated with low birth weight and foetal abnormalities, in addition to cataract and high IOP risk in the mother.
- Anti-VEGF may be associated with foetal problems, and is best avoided due to a lack of safety data in pregnancy.

4.5.4.4 Treatment of Persistent Diabetic Maculopathy

The extent of peripheral retinal nonperfusion correlates with the severity of macular oedema in diabetic retinopathy and vein occlusion. Non-responsive macular oedema should be investigated for peripheral ischaemia by widefield angiography (UWFA).

Objective and quantitative measurement tools using VA, OCT, retinal vascular dynamics on OCT-A (number of microaneurysms, amount and areas of leakage, and quantitative assessment of retinal perfusion), and angiographic parameters, provide objective tools to monitor disease progression and treatment response in DME and RVO (REACT and PERMEATE studies).

Reasons for persistent diabetic maculopathy:
- Suboptimal initial treatment.
- OCT features associated with poor response and worse prognosis.
- **Ischaemic maculopathy.**
- Centre involving CSME – not amenable to laser treatment
- Sub-macular hyperreflective foci seen in OCT is associated with chronicity and worse prognosis.

An FFA or OCT-A will differentiate an exudative from ischaemic maculopathy, where targeted treatment may be helpful. Random, excessive laser should be avoided.
Treatment of persistent diabetic maculopathy – assess CRT on OCT
- If CRT >400 μm – treat with IVT (anti-VEGF).
- Pseudophakes with CRT <400 μm – consider IVTA or Ozurdex implant.
- Phakic patients with CRT <400 μm – watch closely and treat with IVT if worsens.
- **Chronic DMO may respond better to IV steroid.**
- Surgical intervention is necessary in patients with vitreoretinal interface problems like ERM, VMT.
- Ischaemic maculopathy – avoid further laser, poor prognosis.

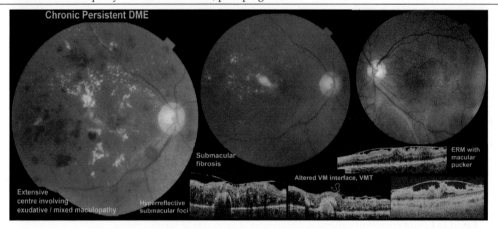

Figure 4.113 Chronic persistent DME.

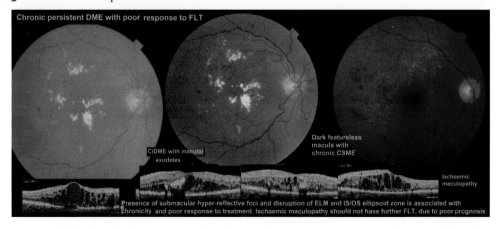

Figure 4.114 Chronic persistent DME – 1.

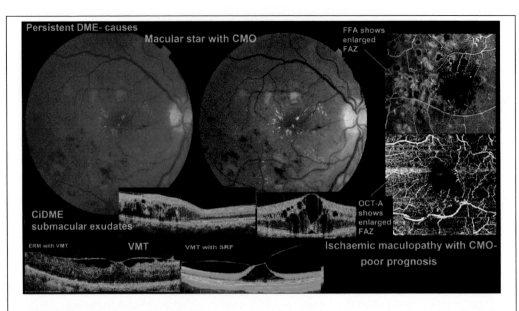

Figure 4.115 Causes of persistent DME.

4.5.4.5 Complications of Laser Treatment

Loss of Vision, Scotoma
- Laser treatment is destructive to RPE and overlying neuro-retina, causing central and paracentral scotomas. They are worse with heavy laser (high power, large spots, and longer pulses) and manifest as heavily pigmented burns.
- Acute visual loss occurs from an inadvertent macular burn.
- Delayed loss occurs from **burn creep – enlargement of laser scar to involve fovea.**

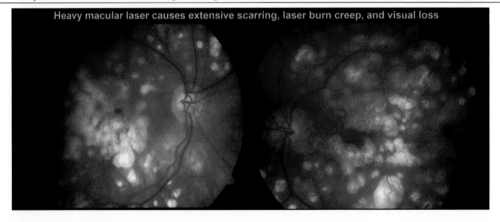

Figure 4.116 Heavy FLT with macular scar.

Other Side Effects
- Floaters (vitreous syneresis) – common, usually settle spontaneously.
- Temporary – eye ache and headache, blurring, colour de-saturation, photophobia.

Choroidal Neovascularization/Iatrogenic CNV
- FLT using high power with an extremely small spot, close to the macula, can lead to break in Bruch's membrane and formation of CNV.
- The risk is higher in pigmented fundi, and with macular haemorrhage, as both pigment and blood strongly absorb laser light, resulting in a deep burn.
- **Reduce power and treat sparingly when working close to the macula.**

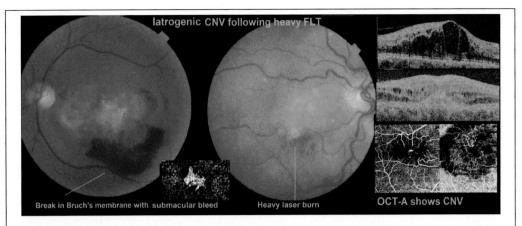

Figure 4.117 Iatrogenic CNV after FLT.

ERM, Macular Pucker
- Excessive FLT causes fibrosis of nearby NVE or worsening of pre-existing ERM.
- Contraction of ERM causes wrinkling and macular distortion, with visual problems, and can lead to lamellar hole or FTMH.
- Pre-existing ERM should be documented with vision and OCT, prior to laser treatment, and patients should have gentle, subthreshold laser treatment, keeping the laser count to minimum, to prevent worsening.
- **A VR referral may be needed in severe cases.**

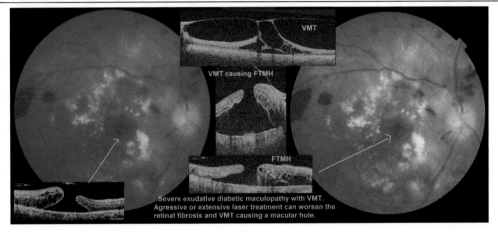

Figure 4.118 Severe DME causing FTMH.

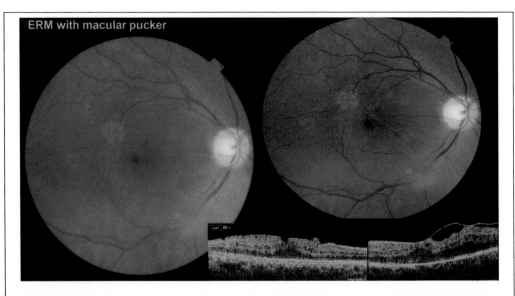

Figure 4.119 ERM with macular pucker.

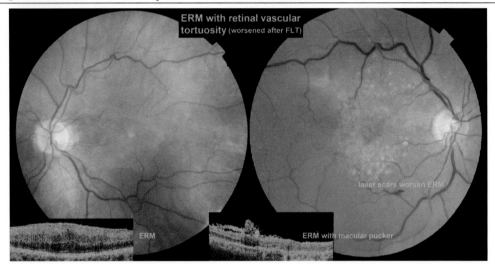

Figure 4.120 ERM worsens after FLT.

SUGGESTED READING

1. *ETDRS Research Group. Techniques for scatter and local laser treatment of DR- report numbers- 2,3,9*

2. The DRS Research Group. Photocoagulation treatment of PDR. Clinical application of DRS findings, report no 8. *Ophthalmology.* 1981;88:583–600.

3. Neubauer, A.S. et al. Laser treatment in DR. *Ophthalmologica.* 2007;221(2):95–102.

4. Lee, C.M. et al. Modied grid laser for diffuse DME. Long-term visual results. *Ophthalmology.* 1991;98(10):1594–1602.

5. Blumenkranz, M.S. et al. Non-damaging photothermal therapy of the retina using EPM semiautomated patterned scanning laser for retinal photocoagulation. *Retina.* 2006;26:370–376.

6. Lock, J.H. et al. An update on retinal laser therapy. *Clin Exp Optom.* 2011;94:43–51.

7. Hariprasad, S.M. et al. New approaches to retinal laser therapy. *Retin Physician.* 2009;6(7):58–61.

4.6 FOCAL LASER TREATMENT FOR NON-DIABETIC MACULOPATHIES

4.6.1 Retinal Vein Occlusion

4.6.1.1 CRVO and HRVO

- **FLT is not beneficial for macular oedema associated with CRVO and HRVO. The first line treatment is IVT.**
- **Phakic patients are treated with anti-VEGF.**
- **Pseudophakic patients are treated with anti-VEGF, IVTA, or steroid implant.**

Although FLT is not helpful, these patients may need PRP (sectoral or total) in the presence of significant ischaemia and neovascularization (*CVOS*).

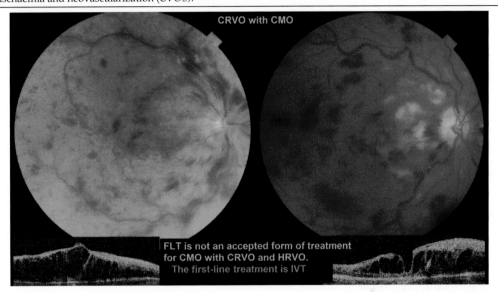

Figure 4.121 CRVO with CMO.

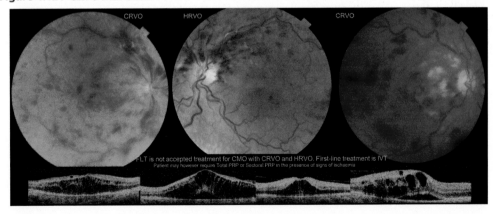

Figure 4.122 FLT not done in CRVO and HRVO.

Hemiretinal Vein Occlusion

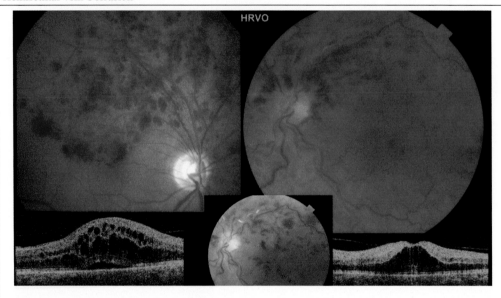

Figure 4.123 HRVO with CMO.

4.6.1.2 *Branch Retinal Vein Occlusion*

The Branch Vein Occlusion Study (BVOS) showed the efficacy of the grid laser in macular oedema secondary to BRVO.

- **OCT** documents the extent of MO, response to treatment, and pre-existing VMT problems.

- **FFA and OCT-A** – help identify area of occlusion, collaterals, new vessels, and decide on appropriate treatment modality, based on the extent of retinal ischaemia.
- If FFA is not available, look closely for collaterals in the perimacular area, around the venous blockage. Collaterals are bypass vessels that re-perfuse the retina and reduce macular oedema in BRVO.
- **Avoid laser damage to collaterals as it will worsen macular oedema and vision.**

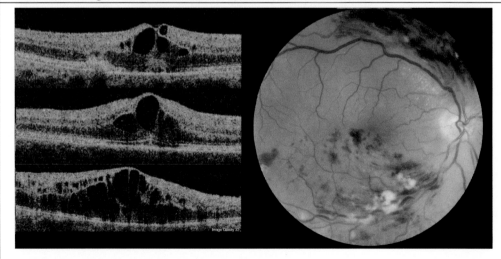

Figure 4.124 BRVO with CMO.

Indication for FLT in BRVO with persistent CMO (>3/12 duration):
- Patient unwilling or unsuitable (due to ill health or socio-economic reason) for IVT, or as an adjunct to IVT, to reduce number of injections.
- **BRVO with extrafoveal exudates or circinate, which are unlikely to shift with IVT.**

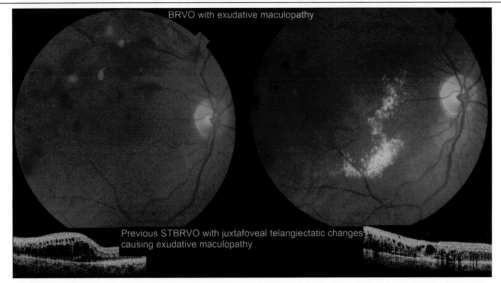

Figure 4.125 STBRVO with exudative maculopathy.

- **Grid laser treatment in BRVO – Select single spot, Mainster focal CL**
- VA< 6/12; BRVO with CMO of > 3-month duration, patient unwilling or unsuitable for IVT
- **Number of shots (grid) – 25–50 × spot size -100μm × pulse duration 10ms × 1 spot gap × power 100–200mw (light grey burns) (higher power in oedematous areas).**
- **Additionally, patients may need sectoral PRP.**

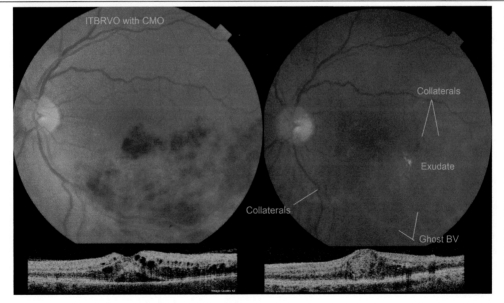

Figure 4.126 ITBRVO with CMO-1.

Collaterals develop and help clear the CMO. FLT is only required if CMO persists.

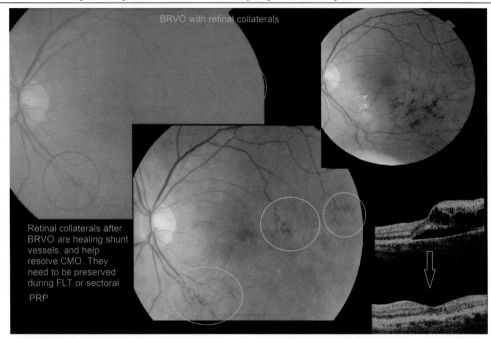

Figure 4.127 ITBRVO with retinal collaterals.

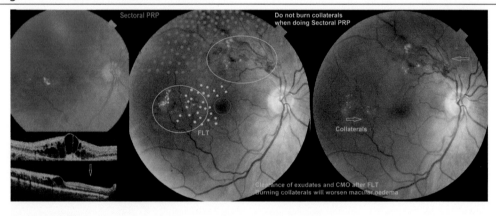

Figure 4.128 BRVO with FLT.

4.6.2 Retinal Artery Macroaneurysm (RAM)

RAM are common in elderly (age >60), female patients with high BP, and atherosclerosis. They may be asymptomatic or present with visual loss or distortion, depending on their location. The clinical course is variable, but most involute spontaneously.

Leakage from a RAM can cause sub-RPE, subretinal, intra-retinal, preretinal, subhyaloid, or vitreous haemorrhages. The involved artery may show proximal and distal narrowing. RAM can cause CMO, macular deposition of hard exudates, ERM, macular holes, and branch retinal artery occlusion. The outcome is poor with sub-macular involvement.

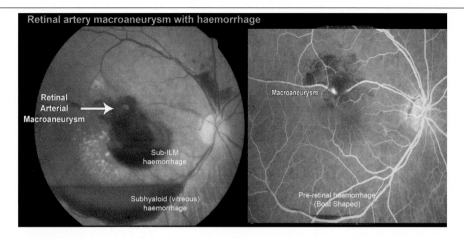

Figure 4.129 RAM with haemorrhage – 1.

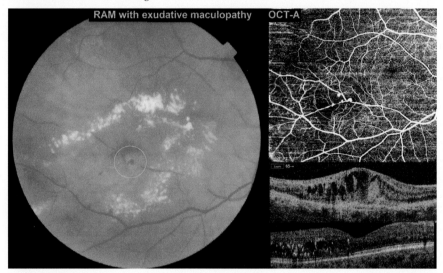

Figure 4.130 RAM with exudative maculopathy.

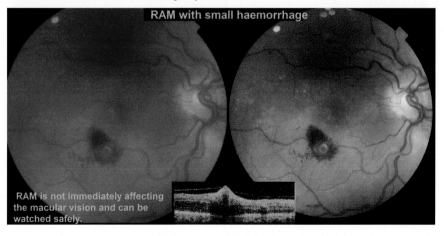

Figure 4.131 RAM with small haemorrhage.

- **If vision (macular area) is not affected, no treatment is required.**
- **Most RAMs will involve and clear up spontaneously (auto infarct).**
- Treatment is only required for exudative or haemorrhagic RAMs, with persistent MO.
- Laser of the artery and surrounding area **decreases blood flow and intraluminal pressure within the RAM**, reducing leakage and causing it to close in 20% of cases.

Anti-VEGF therapy may help by blocking angiogenesis and reducing vascular permeability, to reduce further bleeding and exudation.

Other treatment options include:
- Pneumatic displacement of sub-macular haemorrhages (TPA and gas).
- Pars plana vitrectomy to clear persistent vitreous haemorrhage.
- Sub-macular surgery with tissue plasminogen activator-assisted thrombolysis.

Side Effects of Laser Treatment
- Laser scar creep and subretinal fibrosis causing visual loss and scotoma.
- Branch retinal artery occlusion, CRAO, AV shunt formation.
- Deposition of hard exudates and scarring, as serous fluid is absorbed.
- Pre-retinal haemorrhage or vitreous haemorrhage.
- ERM, macular pucker, VR traction.
- Iatrogenic CNV.

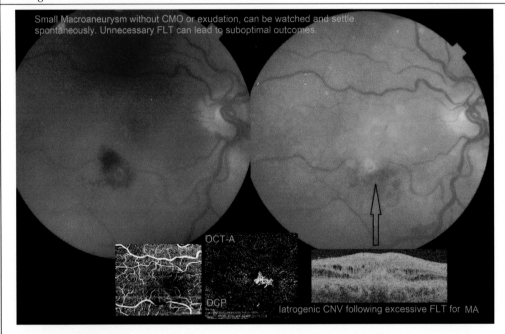

Figure 4.132 Macroaneurysm with iatrogenic CNV.

- **FLT is reserved for patients with sight-threatening problems.**
- 16% to 27% of RAMs are successfully thrombosed following FLT.
- **Direct laser to RAM** should be applied cautiously, with low power, long pulse, and large spot to avoid rupture and arterial occlusion.

- **Indirect FLT around RAM – safer,** reduces blood flow, decreases exudation, and aids closure. This technique reduces risk of arteriolar occlusion and rupture of RAM.

- It is not established which methods are superior, and some physicians prefer a combination of both direct and indirect laser.
- **Threshold versus subthreshold laser** – have comparable visual and anatomical outcomes, with **reduced ERM formation in the subthreshold group.**

Direct laser treatment – with single spot and Mainster Focal CL
- **Spot size – 300–400 µm (large) × pulse duration 20–30 ms (long) × power 200–300 mw (low power to get just visible burns) × number of shots 5–10 shots directly over the aneurysm, confluent burns.**

- **Indirect laser – 10–15 shots around the MA.**
- **200–400 µm spot size × 200–300 mw power × 20–30 ms exposure time.**

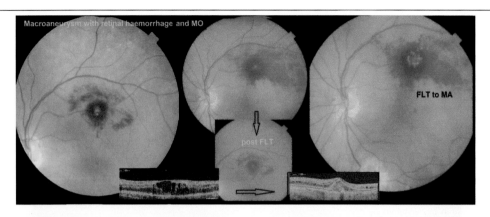

Figure 4.133 Macroaneurysm treated with FLT.

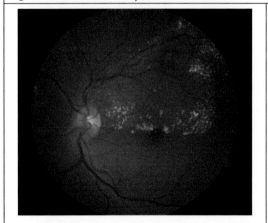

Figure 4.134 RAM with leak.

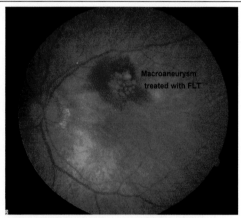

Figure 4.135 RAM treated with FLT.

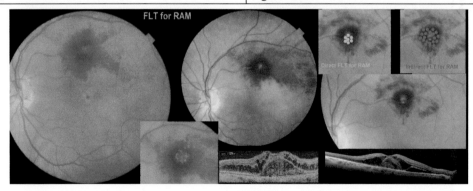

Figure 4.136 FLT for RAM.

4.6.3 Central Serous Chorioretinopathy (CSCR)

CSCR is detachment of the neurosensory retina, with yellowish discolouration at the fovea due to increased visibility of xanthophyll pigment, associated with choroidal and RPE ischaemia, hyperpermeability, and dysfunction. Presentation can be **acute or chronic**, with symptoms of central scotoma, metamorphopsia, dyschromatopsia, micropsia, and hyperopic refractive shift. Loss of RPE cells and failure of RPE pump causes pinpoint leakage in the subretinal space.

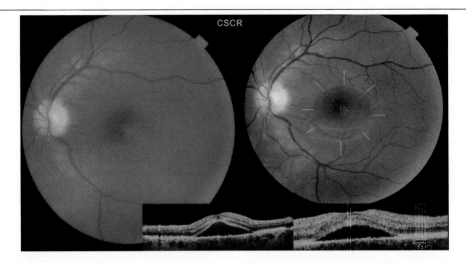

Figure 4.137 CSCR.

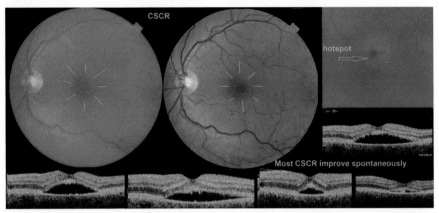

Figure 4.138 CSCR-2.

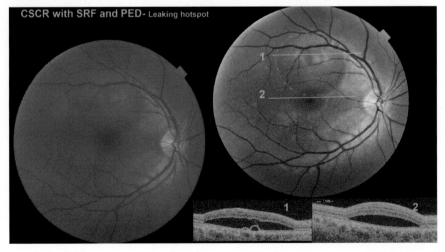

Figure 4.139 CSCR with SRF and extrafoveal PED.

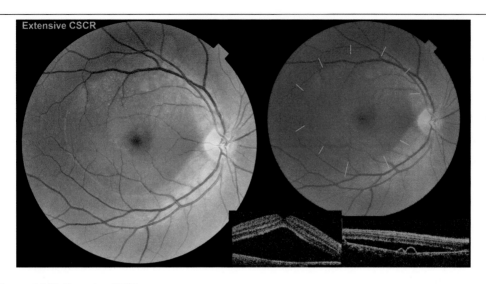

Figure 4.140 Extensive CSCR.

SRF is clear initially, but can turn cloudy in chronic cases, with PED and leaking hotspots. Recurrent, chronic CSCR leads to RPE atrophy, pigmentary changes, and subretinal fibrosis.

- **FFA shows points of leakage with late pooling into the serous detachment,** which can be inkblot or smokestack in appearance.
- **ICG – Indocyanine green angiography** shows focal delay and hyperpermeability in the choroidal circulation.

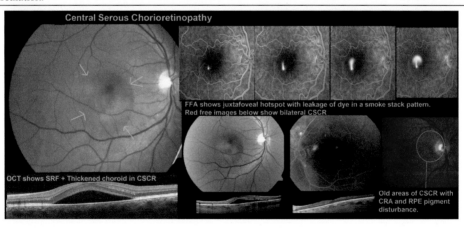

Figure 4.141 CSCR – 1.

OCT demonstrates SRF, with focal PED (pigment epithelial detachment).
SDOCT (enhanced depth imaging) has shown increased sub-foveal choroidal thickness in CSCR.

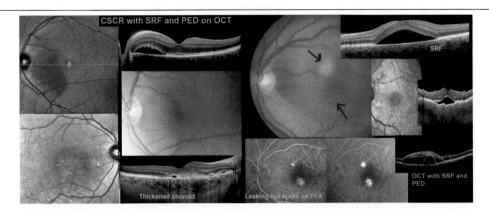

Figure 4.142 CSCR with OCT changes.

- Currently, there is no 'gold standard' treatment for CSCR.

- **Most CSCR are self-limiting (settle spontaneously in 3–4 months), and do not require any active treatment.** Only recurrent or persistent cases require treatment.

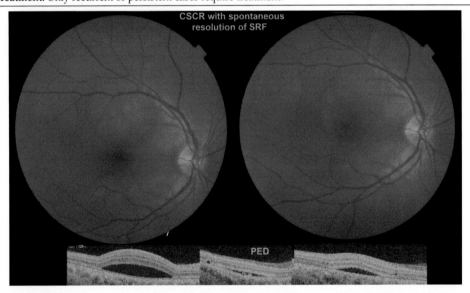

Figure 4.143 CSCR with spontaneous resolution of SRF.

- Recurrent or persistent chronic CSCR, with visual loss, needs an FFA to find the **hot spots (leaking areas). If the hot spots are extrafoveal they can be targeted with gentle macular laser (2–4 burns) directly to the hot spots.**

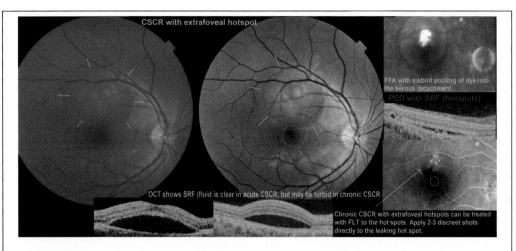

Figure 4.144 CSCR with FLT.

- Laser treatment is not appropriate for juxtafoveal or sub-foveal leakage.

- Laser treatment parameters are the same as FLT using a single spot and Mainster Focal CL.
- 2–4 shots (to leaking hot spots) × 60–100 μm (spot size, depending on proximity to macula) × 10ms (exposure time) × 100–150 mw (power), gentle light grey burn.
- Do not retreat/overtreat the area. Gentle laser stimulates RPE to absorb the fluid.

- CSCR responds well to newer vision sparing, subthreshold, and micro-pulse laser (MPL), effective in treating both extrafoveal and juxtafoveal leakage.

- Risks of treatment include macular burns, central or paracentral scotoma, ERM, macular pucker, iatrogenic CNV, and failure of treatment.

- **Photodynamic treatment (PDT)** has been used for persistent CSCR with some success, but can cause RPE atrophy, choroidal ischaemia, and transient reduction of macular functions. PDT directly targets choroidal circulation and may be used in patients with sub-foveal and multifocal points of leakage.

4.6.4 Idiopathic Juxtafoveal Telangiectasia (IJFT)

IJFT are unilateral or bilateral alterations of parafoveal capillary network, causing macular oedema, exudation, and scarring. Symptoms vary from being asymptomatic, mild visual disturbances, metamorphopsia, and scotomas to progressive visual loss.

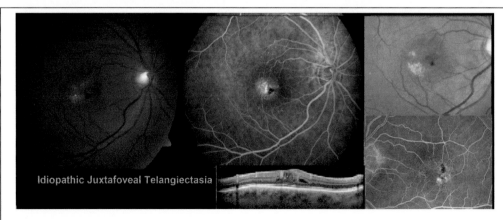

Figure 4.145 IJFT.

They are classified into three types:

Type I – congenital, unilateral, visible telangiectasis, common in males, visual loss due to CMO.

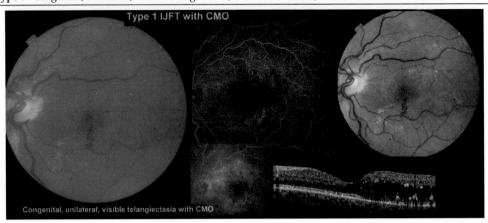

Figure 4.146 Type 1 IJFT.

Type II – commonest, acquired, bilateral, in middle-aged patients, telangiectasis not obvious clinically, but seen on OCT and FFA. Visual loss is due to retinal atrophy (not exudation), and subretinal neovascularization is common.
Progresses through five stages – stages 1–4 are non-proliferative, with telangiectasis and foveal atrophy. Stage 5 is a proliferative stage, associated with subretinal exudates, crystals, haemorrhage, RPE pigment migration, retino-choroidal anastomosis, and SR-CNV.

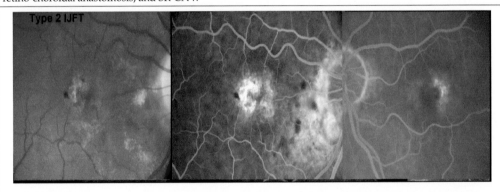

Figure 4.147 Type 2 IJFT.

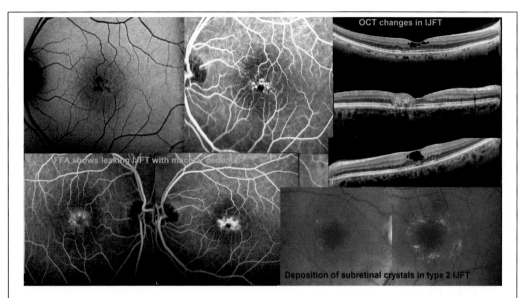

Figure 4.148 Type 2 IJFT – 1.

Type III – rare, characterized by progressive obliteration of perifoveal capillary network, often associated with a medical or neurologic disease.

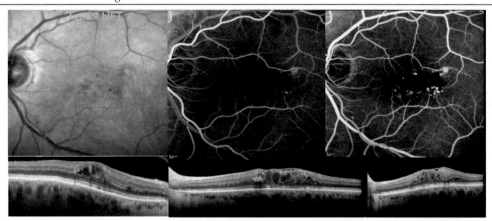

Figure 4.149 Type 3 IJFT.

Treatment to reduce leakage and exudation and stabilize MO and vision includes:
- Laser photocoagulation.
- IV anti-VEGF.
- IV steroids (IVTA) – stabilizes blood-retinal barrier and reduces VEGF production, but the effect is short-lived and the side-effect profile limits its use.

Photocoagulation should be used sparingly to reduce the risk of paracentral scotoma, metamorphopsia, and iatrogenic CNV.

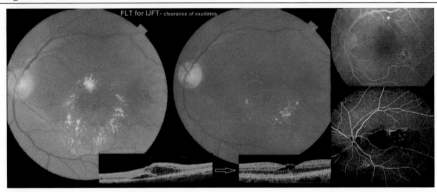

Figure 4.150 FLT for IJFT – clearance of exudates.

Laser Treatment
- **Single shot selection**
- **5–15 shots × 100 μm spot size × 10 ms exposure time × 120–200 mw power × Mainster Focal lens – target individual leaking telangiectatic vessels.**
- **Multiple treatment sessions with small treatment areas are preferred.**
- **It is not necessary to destroy every dilated capillary, and initial treatment should avoid telangiectasia close to the FAZ.**

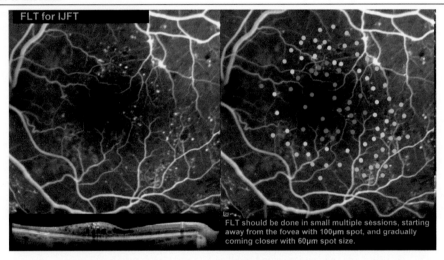

Figure 4.151 FLT for IJFT.

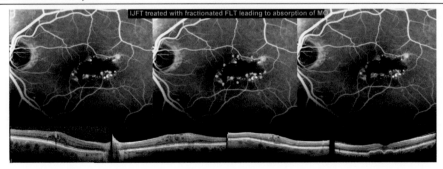

Figure 4.152 IJFT treated with FLT.

4.6.5 Laser Treatment for Age Related Macular Degeneration

First-line treatment for wet ARMD is intravitreal anti-VEGF injections.

Although laser may be beneficial in certain patients, it is no longer the preferred treatment.

- **Laser treatment** used to destroy extrafoveal CNV was associated with scarring, visual loss, and development of scotoma, with **a high risk of sub-foveal extension of CNV, and significant visual loss. It is no longer done for AMD maculopathy.**
- **There is renewed interest in laser treatment with the new MPL and NPL,** which can slow progression of AMD and restore RPE function.
- **Subthreshold MPL (SDM) may re-sensitize RPE in wet AMD unresponsive to anti-VEGF therapy in 90% of cases.**

Photodynamic Therapy (PDT) with Diode
- A light-sensitive dye (Visudyne) injected intravenously accumulates in the CNV membrane. A diode laser activates the dye, inducing phototoxic effects to clot the vessels. As the injected dye collects in the blood vessels of the choroidal neovascular membrane, PDT spares the central foveal avascular zone.
- **PDT is useful in treating retinal polyps, which do not respond as well to anti-VEGF injections.**

4.7 LASER RETINOPEXY

Retinal holes and tears are often encountered during routine fundoscopy and pose a risk for retinal detachment. A symptomatic retinal tear presents with a sudden onset of flashing lights (photopsia), floaters, blurred vision, or visual field loss, due to vitreous haemorrhage or retinal detachment.

Common risk factors include myopia, aphakia, ocular surgery, trauma, detachment in the fellow eye, and family history. Peripheral retinal degenerations are associated with an increased risk of recurrent tears and detachment.

4.7.1 Peripheral Retinal Degenerations

Peripheral retinal degenerations typically occur between the equator and ora-serrata. Some changes may only be apparent with scleral depression.

Vitreoretinal degeneration **High risk of holes/tears**	Intraretinal degeneration **Low risk of tears/holes**	Chorioretinal degeneration **No risk of tears/holes**
Lattice degeneration Snail track degeneration Snowflake degeneration White without pressure (WWOP) Tractional tuft	Micro-cystoid degeneration (typical and reticular) Degenerative Retinoschisis Pars plana cyst	Paving stone degeneration Honeycomb degeneration Peripheral drusen

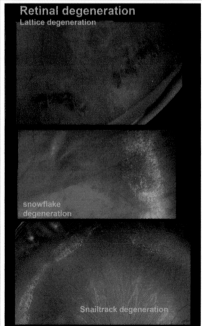

	Lattice Degeneration Commonest (7–8% of population), familial predilection, common in myopes, unilateral or bilateral (40–50%), appear as areas of retinal thinning, with arborizing network of white or pigmented lines crossing blood vessels. They are associated with vitreous liquefaction, atrophic holes with VR adhesions, high risk of tear or RD following an acute PVD. 25% of patients with RD had lattice degeneration, of which 83% had the tear within an area of lattice.
	Snail Track Degeneration Sharply demarcated, elongated bands of white frost-like inner retinal changes, mimicking a snail track. Thought to be precursors to lattice degeneration. Often bilateral, in ST quadrant of young myopes, frequently associated with atrophic round holes with VR traction.
	Snowflake Degeneration Multiple glistening yellow white dots scattered diffusely in peripheral fundus. Associated with fibrillar vitreous degeneration, cataracts, and corneal guttata.

Figure 4.153 Retinal degeneration.

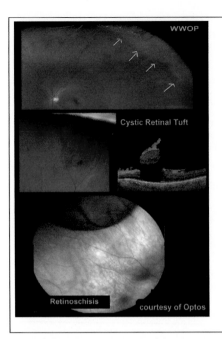

White without Pressure Greyish-white peripheral retina with a well-demarcated border, due to reduced blood flow in the area, with VR traction. Common in elderly myopes, may cause giant retinal tears and RD.
Cystic Retinal Tufts Congenital round, white tuft composed of glial tissue with surface vitreous condensation and pigmentary changes. The incidence of RD from a cystic retinal tuft is approximately 0.28%.
Degenerative Retinoschisis Split in retina, bilateral (70–80%), symmetrical, commonly involving IT quadrant, immobile dome-shaped elevation of inner retinal layer, with surface snowflakes, micro-cystoid changes and vascular sheathing. Rarely, causes RD (<2.5%) with a break in both layers of the schisis. Two forms – **typical** (split in outer plexiform layer) and **reticular** (split in NFL), causes absolute scotoma.

4.7.2 Diagnosis of Retinal Holes and Tears

Retinal holes appear on fundal examination (90D, 3-mirror lens, or BIO with indentation) as a round, red lesion (increased glow from underlying choriocapillaris), sometimes with a cuff of SRF, representing a localized detachment. An operculated hole will show an overlying operculum.

4.7.3 Role of Posterior Vitreous Detachment

The commonest event preceding a full-thickness retinal break is a PVD with flashing lights and floaters. PVD associated with peripheral retinal degenerations have a higher risk of developing tears and patients should be warned of the risk.

Symptomatic PVD without retinal breaks require no immediate treatment but need re-examination within 2 weeks, as breaks may develop later. When examining patients with acute PVD, the presence or absence of pigment (tobacco dust or Shafer's sign) or red blood cells consistent with a vitreous haemorrhage is important to confirm or rule out a retinal tear.

4.7.4 Formation of Retinal Holes and Tears

Atrophic retinal holes (5% of routine fundal examination) tend to be asymptomatic.

- Due to progressive retinal thinning associated with retinal degeneration (not VRT).
- Frequently associated with lattice degeneration, with a cuff of SRF (liquefaction of overlying vitreous) or abnormal vitreoretinal adhesions at the edges; have a 7% chance of developing RD following a PVD.

- There is no clear consensus on treatment, and most can be monitored. Treatment is reserved for high-risk patients (**vitreoretinal disease, high myopia, occupation [boxer], contact sports, family history of RD, detachment in fellow eye, and prior to intraocular surgery**).

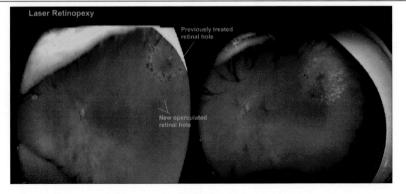

Figure 4.154 Laser retinopexy for atrophic retinal hole.

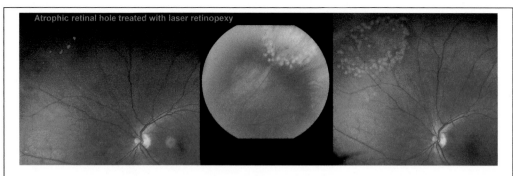

Figure 4.155 Laser retinopexy for atrophic retinal hole.

4.7.5 Operculated Retinal Holes

- Operculated holes usually originate in areas of vitreoretinal tufts with a weak underlying retina. Trauma or PVD causes avulsion of the tuft, leading to a full-thickness hole with an overlying operculum.
- Laser treatment is advised for an operculated hole to prevent RD.

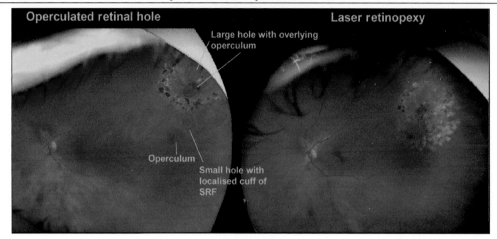

Figure 4.156 Retinopexy for operculated retinal hole with SRF.

4.7.6 Horseshoe Tear

Horseshoe tear is the commonest cause of RD, following PVD, with associated risk factors (aging, myopia, lattice degeneration, and trauma). The flap is attached to the retina but can be completely avulsed creating a floating operculum. Associated with a high risk of RD and should be treated with urgent retinopexy.

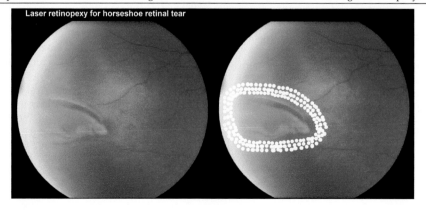

Figure 4.157 Laser retinopexy for horseshoe retinal tear.

Giant Retinal Tears and Retinal Dialysis
- Giant tears extend more than three-clock hours, and retinal dialysis is a break at the ora serrata following trauma, generally in young patients with strong vitreous attachments.
- Both conditions pose management challenges and are not amenable to laser treatment. They need surgical intervention including vitrectomy with gas or oil, scleral buckle, and endo-laser or cryotherapy.

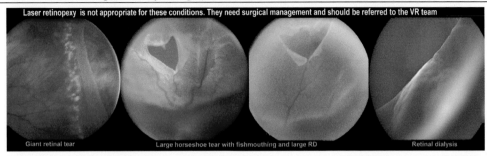

Laser retinopexy is not appropriate for these conditions. They need surgical management and should be referred to the VR team

Giant retinal tear · Large horseshoe tear with fishmouthing and large RD · Retinal dialysis

Figure 4.158 Laser retinopexy is not appropriate for these conditions.

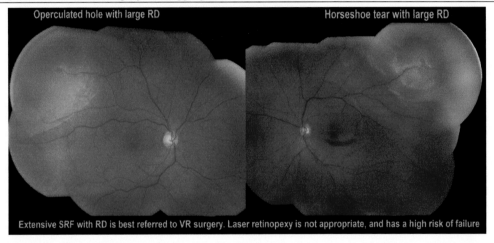

Operculated hole with large RD · Horseshoe tear with large RD

Extensive SRF with RD is best referred to VR surgery. Laser retinopexy is not appropriate, and has a high risk of failure

Figure 4.159 Retinal tears with RD.

4.7.7 Treatment of Retinal Holes and Tears

Retinopexy involves scarification of the retina and RPE with laser photocoagulation, diathermy, or cryotherapy, creating strong adhesion between retina and RPE, to seal the tear and prevent a retinal detachment.

All forms of retinopexy create tissue destruction, scarring, and further VR traction, and should be used as little as possible. Continuous laser is preferable to intermittent laser because it causes uniform tissue destruction, resulting in uniform retinal tissue tensile strength, reducing the risk of traction elsewhere.

All forms of retinopexy are effective, but laser photocoagulation and diathermy are preferable for a rapid bond development. Laser photocoagulation produces bonds approaching normal strength within 24 hours, from local effects such as fibrin formation, and double the normal strength by 2–3 weeks after photocoagulation. Cryotherapy weakens adhesion in the first week (due to inflammation and oedema), after which adhesive force rises to the same levels as other forms of retinopexy, and is preferred for more anterior lesions.

With laser photocoagulation, a significant number of patients require further intervention, due to inadequate coverage of the break or presence of SRF affecting outcome.

4.7.8 Laser Retinopexy – Procedure

Pre-treatment
- The aim is to prevent the development of retinal detachment.
- Patients are warned of the risk of retinal detachment despite treatment, especially in the presence of lattice degeneration, traumatic tears, inadequately treated holes/tears, or those associated with localised RD (cuff of SRF).
- **Ensure pupils are maximally dilated** (tropicamide + phenylepherine × 2) to make retinopexy safe and easy to complete.

- **Contact lens** with topical anaesthesia and coupling lubricant – **selected based on location of the tear.**

Mid-peripheral tear – Mainster ×1 lens or 3-mirror (broad mirror)

Far peripheral tear – select one of these three lenses:

If pupil is well dilated use 3-mirror lens (orientate tall mirror opposite to tear) – this offers higher magnification and better visualization.

Mainster-165 wide field lens	Wide FOV, lower magnification, difficulty seeing hole, and laser burns
QuadrAspheric Lens (small pupils, small PA)	

Slit lamp settings – same as PRP
- **Use low magnification (×6) to allow wide FOV.**

Select laser parameters
- Select posterior treatment, pattern option – 2×2 square grid.
- Spot size – 200μm (pre-set); exposure time – 20ms (pre-set).
- Reduce spot gap to zero – confluent burns.
- Power – start at 300mw and titrate up to get white burns.
- Go all around the hole/tear, with 2 rows of 2×2 confluent burns (four rows around the hole).
- You can use single spot (200um) and do three rows of confluent burns around the hole. This takes a little bit longer than the 2×2 grid.

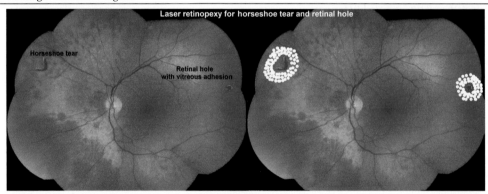

Figure 4.160 Laser retinopexy for horseshoe tear and retinal hole.

PASCAL Retinopexy Patterns
- PASCAL has pre-selected patterns (arcs and circles) for retinopexy, which can be placed around the tear and deliver multiple shots in one go.
- The diameter of the circle can be altered to size, or a series of arcs placed around the hole using a rotate/advance pattern to complete treatment.
- **Although these seem advantageous to use, they are effectively less controlled ways of performing a retinopexy.**
  - Multiple shots are painful, take longer to deliver, and early release of the foot pedal may result in incomplete delivery of the pattern.
  - Eye or head movements can deliver patterns in the wrong areas.
  - A large pattern generates glare during treatment, making visualization difficult.
  - Large grids are difficult to focus precisely peripherally.

The best way to do a retinopexy is under direct, constant view, using a small 2×2 confluent grid, with a 3-mirror lens.

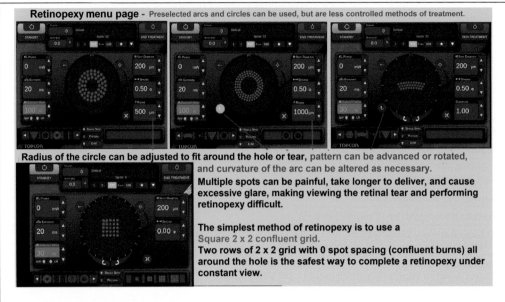

Figure 4.161 Laser retinopexy menu page.

4.7.9 Special Situations

Retinal Tears with Localized RD
- Can be lasered if the RD is less than 2–3 clock hours.
- Larger RD should be referred for VR surgery.
- Laser uptake over SRF may be poor, with risk of treatment failure and progression.
- Consider **posturing patient for an hour** before treatment, to allow drainage of SRF, making laser easier. (Keep location of tear lowest, relative to other parts of the body).
- If the tear is associated with a small cuff of SRF, the easiest option is to go directly around the SRF (wider area of treatment, more shots).
- Higher power and increased pulse duration may be required as uptake may be poor in presence of SRF.
- Watch closely – risk of RD is high, even after treatment.

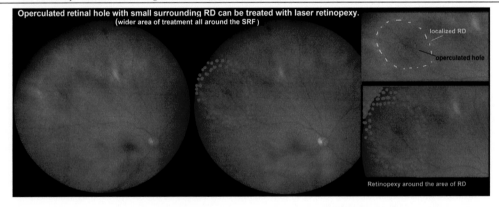

Figure 4.162 Laser retinopexy for operculated retinal hole with localized RD.

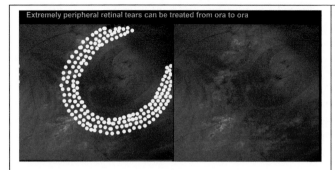

Figure 4.163 Extremely peripheral tear.

Extremely peripheral holes and tears may not have enough room at the anterior edge to complete a retinopexy. **Lasering from ora to ora is acceptable, provided the patient is warned of RD risk. Alternatively, they can be referred for treatment with cryotherapy.**

Lattice Degeneration with Retinal Holes and Tears
- Lattice degeneration represents areas of weakness on the retina. Heavy laser in one area causes scarring, creating traction in an adjacent area, with the risk of developing a new tear. Low-risk lattice degeneration with small atrophic holes may be watched rather than treated. When lasering patients with lattice degeneration, extreme caution must be exercised, using low power and minimum number of shots.
- **NEVER LASER A LATTICE DIRECTLY – it may induce a tear.**
- **DO NOT LASER HEAVILY around a lattice.**
- **A hole/tear associated with a lattice needs treatment all around the lattice area, not just the hole.**

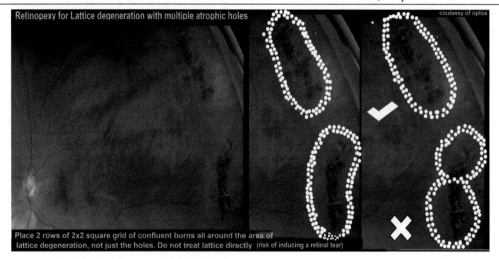

Figure 4.164 Retinopexy with lattice degeneration.

Prophylactic treatment of lattice is not indicated, except with high-risk associations. **Excessive laser, in the presence of lattice degeneration, creates unnecessary VRT and may induce a retinal hole or tear elsewhere.**
- **Low-risk patients** – small atrophic holes, with no vitreous adhesions, inferior quadrant, patient not myopic, no previous history or family history of tears/RD, do not need laser treatment and can be watched with warning signs of RD.
- **High-risk patients** – superior quadrant, multiple holes, vitreous adhesions, high myope, extensive lattice, previous history, or family history of RD, contact sports (boxing, rugby) require treatment.

SUGGESTED READING

1. Kim, B.Y et al. OCT patterns of DME. *Am J Ophthalmol.* 2006;142:405–412.

2. Otani, T. et al. Patterns of DME with OCT. *Am J Ophthalmol.* 1999;127:688–693.

3. De Carlo, T.E. et al. A review of OCT-A. *Int J Retina Vitreous.* 2015;1:5.

4. Maheshwary, A.S. et al. Association between percent disruption of photoreceptor IS-OS junction and VA in DME. *Am J Ophth.* 2010;150(1):63–67. doi: 10.1016/j.ajo.2010.01.039. Epub 2010 May 10.

5. Kang, J.W. et al. Correlation of OCT hyperreflective foci with visual outcomes in DME. *Retina.* 2016;36:1630–1639.

6. Phadikar, P. et al. The potential of SD-OCT imaging based retinal biomarkers. *Int J Retina Vitreous*. 2017;3:1–10.

7. Yadav, N.K. et al. Recent developments in retinal lasers and delivery systems. *Ind J Ophthalmol*. 2014;62:50–54.

8. Wessel, M.M. et al. Peripheral retinal ischemia, by UWFA, is associated with DME. *BJO*. 2012;96:694–698.

9. Kim, N.R. et al. OCT patterns in DME: prediction of visual outcome after FLT. *BJO*. 2009;93(7):901–905.

10. Ghazi, N.G. et al. OCT findings in persistent DME: vitreomacular interface. *Am J Ophthalmol*.2007;144:747–754.

11. Pedinielli, A. et al. Three different OCT-A measurement methods to assess capillary density changes in DR. *Ophthalmic Surg Lasers Imaging Retina*. 48:378–384.

12. Hasegawa, N. et al. new insights into mA in DCP detected by OCT-A in DME. *Invest Ophthal Vis Sci*. 2016;57(Oct):348–355.

13. Wessel, M.M. et al. UWFA improves detection and classification of DR. *Retina*. 2012;32:785–791.

14. Oliver, S.C.N. et al. Peripheral vessel leakage (PVL): a new angiographic finding in DR identified with UWFA. *Sem Ophthalmol*. 2010; 25:27–33.

15. BVOS Group. Argon laser photocoagulation for MO in BRVO. *Am J Ophthalmol*. 1984;98(3):271–282.

16. Malik, K.J. et al. Low-intensity/high-density SDM laser for CSCR. *Retina*. 2015.

17. Wang, M. et al. CSCR. *Acta Ophthalmol*. 2008; 86:126–145.

18. Chan, W.M. et al. Treatment of CNV in CSR by PDT. *Am J Ophthalmol*. 2003; 136:836–845.

19. Parodi, M.B. et al. Subthreshold vs threshold Laser for RAM. *Invest Ophth Vis Sci*. 2012;53(4):1783–1786.

20. Gass, J.D. et al. IJFT. Update of classification and follow-up study. *Ophthalmology*. 1993;100:1536–1546.

21. Yannuzzi, L.A et al. Idiopathic macular telangiectasia. *Arch Ophthalmol*. 2006;124:450–460.

22. Charbel, I. P. et al. Macular telangiectasia type 2. *Progr Retin Eye Res*. 2013;34:49–77.

23. Park, D.W. et al. Grid laser photocoagulation for MO in bilateral IJFT. *Ophthalmology*. 1997;104:1838–1846.

24. Luttrull, J.K. et al. Laser re-sensitization of medically unresponsive nARMD: Efficacy and implications. *Retina*. 2015; 35:1184–1194.

25. Blindbaek, S. et al. Prophylactic treatment of retinal breaks--a systematic review. *Acta Ophthalmol*.2015;93(1):3–8.

26. Yoon, Y. et al. Rapid enhancement of retinal adhesion by photocoagulation. *Ophthalmology*. 1988;95:1385–1388.

27. Byer, N.E. Cystic retinal tufts and their relationship to RD. *Arch Ophthalmol*. 1981;99(10):1788–1790.

28. van Overdam, K.A. et al. Symptoms predictive for later development of retinal breaks. *Arch Ophthalmol*. 2001;119(10):1483–1486.

Section 5 Approach to Retinal Vascular Disease

This section clarifies understanding of retinal vascular diseases and an approach to managing these conditions with novel agents and therapies, in a multimodal way to target multiple disease pathways. Treatment strategies used in a synergistic manner improve safety, outcomes, and long-term treatment burden.

5.1 MULTIMODAL TREATMENT OF RETINAL VASCULAR DISEASE

Retinal vascular diseases are complex conditions with multifactorial etiology and pathogenesis. Disease chronicity causes visual disability and poor QoL in the working age population, and is increasingly overwhelming healthcare systems. Newer, efficacious strategies are required for optimal disease management, to improve outcomes and reduce treatment burden.

Since ETDRS (1985), treatment options have changed significantly, backed by RCTs. Novel agents and therapies offer improved safety, efficacy, and synergy, and a multimodal approach targets multiple pathways involved in disease pathogenesis.

Management of diabetic eye disease is challenging, due to persistent or refractory DME, irreversible destructive effects of laser with suboptimal outcomes, intensive schedule of IVT, and regular follow-ups needed for long-term maintenance of vision.

Improved understanding of disease mechanisms, laser-tissue interaction, and technological advances in imaging and treatment have led to rethinking treatment strategies. Identifying disease pathways allows targeted treatment and reduces side-effects, and combination therapy for synergistic effects is redefining standards of care in retinal vascular conditions.

Treatment concepts have shifted from isolated laser treatment to combination therapies that can be tailored to patient's needs in a flexible manner. The most effective shift is use of anti-VEGF agents, either alone or in combination with laser treatment.

Vascular endothelial growth factor (VEGF) plays a key role in hypoxia-mediated macular oedema and retinal neovascularization, causing poor visual outcomes. Anti-VEGF agents have revolutionized management, reducing macular oedema, stabilizing and regressing new vessels, aiding absorption of vitreous haemorrhage, preventing rubeosis, and reducing laser-associated worsening of DME and scarring. Using these agents reduces laser burden and laser-related problems and improves visual outcomes.

Treatment options for retinal vascular diseases include:

- Laser treatment alone.

- Anti-VEGF alone.

- IV steroid injections or implants alone.

- Laser + anti-VEGF combination therapy.

- Laser + steroid combination therapy

- Laser + anti-VEGF + steroid combination therapy

- Laser + surgery – vitrectomy, clearance of vitreous haemorrhage, ERM peel.

- Newer laser treatment – multi spot, subthreshold.

A combination of treatments can work synergistically at various stages of the vascular disease and is the preferred approach. Without anti-VEGF or laser, 10% of patients lose vision each year (ETDRS).

5.1.1 Anti-VEGF Agents Used Alone or in Combination

Anti-VEGF agents are the gold standard treatment for CiDME with CRT >400μm. They are vision sparing, with better outcomes than laser treatment. Common agents are ranibizumab, bevacizumab and aflibercept, with a mean duration of action of 4–8 weeks.

Laser is less effective with significant oedema (CRT >400 μm), requiring extensive treatment, causing excessive scarring.

Laser is not the preferred treatment with significant macular oedema.

Anti-VEGF treatment, though effective, needs frequent monitoring and re-treatment, with potential ocular and systemic side-effects with each treatment. IVT can cause decreased retinal perfusion, CR atrophy, and TRD in patients with florid PDR. The ongoing nature of treatment leads to increased socio-economic costs and medical burden.

A combination strategy is useful, where laser adds a more permanent benefit following an initial course of IVT. Deferred laser treatment is less intensive and reduces the number of injections required in the future. Several studies have explored this combination regime for efficacy, safety, and frequency of treatment. Additionally, anti-VEGFs are effective with fluid and not exudates. Patients with an exudative maculopathy will need laser treatment.

- **The Ride and Rise study confirmed benefits of early treatment in DME >300 μm,** and worse outcome with delay in treatment.
- Laser treatment takes time to show effect (3–6 months), which may represent a delay in optimal treatment. It is advisable to start treatment with anti-VEGF if appropriate and continue IVT, even after deferred laser, for optimal long-term management.

Several RCTs have confirmed the benefits of anti-VEGF in improving vision sustainably.
- **The READ 2 and READ 3 studies** confirmed the favourable initial response but found CRT increased with a longer follow-up. Macular laser treatment helped achieve a more sustained CRT reduction, suggesting that anti-VEGF followed by FLT may be an effective way of reducing frequency of injections, while maintaining vision.

- **DRCR.net Protocol I – combined therapy with deferred laser had a better outcome and avoided additional laser for at least 5 years in 50% of cases.**
- **DRCR.net Protocol S** – ranibizumab monotherapy was as effective as PRP at 2 years.
- **CLARITY study** – aflibercept monotherapy delivered better one-year visual outcomes, compared to PRP.

Overview of RCTs with anti-VEGF

Ranibizumab (Lucentis)	Aflibercept (Eylea)	Bevacizumab (Avastin)	Brolicizumab (Beovue)
READ 2 and 3 study. Resolve study. DRCR.net Protocol-I Restore & Reveal Ride and Rise study Lucidate study	Da-Vinci study Vivid and Vista study (significant anatomical and functional benefits vs laser)	DRCR.net study Protocol H Bolt study (Avastin is currently not approved but used off-label, due to affordability)	Kite and Kestrel Hawk and Harrier study (currently not approved for DME)

Protocol-T of DRCR.net
- The Diabetic Retinopathy Clinical Research Network (**DRCR.net**) Protocol T revealed all three anti-VEGF agents (bevacizumab, ranibizumab and aflibercept) were equally effective in treating DME with good vision.
- **Eylea performed better in patients whose baseline vision was <69 letters.**
- **Based on this, Eylea is preferred in chronic DME, with poor baseline vision.**

Anti-VEGFs (alone or combination) used in PDR has results on par with PRP treatment. They are not commonly used for socio-economic reasons. They can, however, be used to prevent neovascular changes, and clear vitreous haemorrhage, to allow laser delivery.

IVT offers initial protection against neovascularization, but as treatment shifts to T&E, with longer intervals, the protective effect wears off and an ischaemic CRVO or DR can develop rubeosis. It is vital to be aware and consider laser treatment in conjunction with IVT to prevent rubeosis in such patients.

5.1.2 What's 'Visually Significant' DME?

ETDRS described CSME based on clinical findings. Advanced imaging technology has allowed early detection of subtle DME, often before decline in visual functions. **Protocol V** suggested that treatment-naïve patients with CiDME and good vision (20/25 or better) can be managed with observation and follow-up, and treatment criteria are visual acuity-based. However, ideal study conditions do not always reflect the real-world scenario, making assessments and treatment decisions tricky.

5.1.3 Real-World Implications of Visual Assessment

- **Clinic vision is variable** (depending on test techniques, conditions, and motivation).

- **Other factors impact vision** – cataract, ocular surface disease, glaucoma.

- **Fluctuations in diabetic control affect vision.**

- **Progressive disease** – worsening of DME (on OCT), or DR, with good vision.

- **Follow-up intervals are less frequent**, and most patients are not treatment naïve.

5.1.4 Steroids + Laser

Inflammation plays an important role in angiogenesis, vascular hyperpermeability, and pathogenesis of macular oedema in DM and RVO. Steroids down-regulate inflammatory pathways, offering long-term improvement, in combination with laser or anti-VEGF.

Clinical trials have investigated steroids in combination with laser in DME, with positive outcomes in efficacy and longevity (greater reduction of CRT for longer periods) compared to laser or IVT alone, suggesting a synergic response.

Intravitreal Triamcinolone Acetonide (IVTA) – Not Preferred Treatment
- Shorter lasting, requiring repeat injection, 33% risk of IOP rise >10mm Hg, cataract surgery rate was 83% at 3 years, compared to 31% with laser treatment.
- **Protocol B (DRCR.net study) – FLT superior to IVTA.**
- **Protocol I (DRCR.net study) –** showed RBZ + deferred/ prompt laser was better than IVTA + laser, over a 3-year period (except in pseudophakes).
- Trial of suprachoroidal corticosteroid delivery +/– aflibercept currently being done.

Dexamethasone Implant 0.7mg (Ozurdex)
Sustained release implants, reduces need for frequent injections.
- **Mead study** – showed cataract incidence (67.9%) and IOP rise (27.7%).
- **The Ozurdex PLACID study** – showed dexa + laser was better than sham + laser.
- **Bevordex study** – compared **Ozurdex vs Avastin in DME.**
- **Ozurdex Champlain study** – Ozurdex in DME after vitrectomy.

Fluocinolone Acetonide Implant – Retisert, Iluvien
Reduces burden of monthly treatment, in patients with co-morbidities, poor response to anti-VEGF, and refractory DME.
- **Retisert** – improved visual and anatomic outcomes but had high rates of cataract progression (91%) and elevated IOP (61.4% with IOP ≥30 mm Hg).
- **Iluvien – FAME A and FAME B study.** Chronic DME (≥ 3-year duration) had better response than non-chronic DME.

Steroids are useful in pseudophakic and aphakic patients with poor response to anti-VEGF agents, chronic refractory DME, DME following vitrectomy (anti-VEGFs do not stay long in a vitrectomized eye), **CMO with CRVO, and systemic vascular comorbidities that preclude use of anti-VEGF agents.**

Steroid use, however, is limited by a high risk of adverse events, like IOP elevation needing treatment, formation and progression of cataract requiring surgery, potential retinal toxicity, and anterior migration of implant causing corneal toxicity and oedema.

Steroid implants should be avoided in patients with glaucoma, pseudophakes who have had YAG capsulotomy, PCR, YAG PI, vitrectomy, or zonular dehiscence.

5.1.4.1 Therapy Switching

Protocol I (DRCR.net) concluded that visual response at 12 weeks (3-loading doses), was predictive of the long-term response. So, if the initial response is suboptimal, therapy switch (change to aflibercept, or to steroids) is reasonable. **Early switch (at 3 months) prevents chronicity and achieves better anatomical and visual outcomes.**

5.1.4.2 Lost to Follow-up Patients (LTFU)

Although anti-VEGFs offers better results, they work on a regular, ongoing schedule, and are not ideal in LTFU patients. After LTFU, both groups (laser and IVT) worsen significantly, but the anti-VEGF group had a higher risk of TRD (20%), VMT, and NVG. LTFU patients are better treated with aggressive laser, due to its longer lasting, permanent effect.

5.1.4.3 Surgery

IV Avastin (Bevacizumab) can help clear vitreous haemorrhage to allow PRP and reduce need for vitrectomy (30%). Early vitrectomy, with anti-VEGF prior to surgery, offers better outcomes, with reduced risk of TRD or rebleeds, in persistent (>6/52) vitreous bleeds.

Vitrectomy removes angiogenic growth factors, VMT, posterior hyaloid face (scaffold for NV), and improves transvitreal oxygenation. It is useful in:

- Persistent florid PDR, with poor response or no further room to laser.

- DME refractory to IVT (often with abnormal VM interface).

- Persistent vitreous haemorrhage (>6 weeks).

- TRD, tractional macular detachment, fibrous membranes affecting vision.

- Macular hole, macular pucker, sub-macular, or retro-hyaloid haemorrhage.

5.1.4.4 Cataract Surgery

Diabetic eye disease is known to worsen after cataract surgery, and should be stabilized (IVT and laser) prior to surgery. A steroid implant can be used in perioperative DME (inflammatory pathways are more relevant after surgery). The post-operative period requires close monitoring for progression and treatment of DR.

Future direction – new treatments (phase 1 or 2 trials) for safety and efficacy in DME.

- READ-4 study (RBZ and tocilizumab – an interleukin-6 inhibitor).
- VIDI study – (ASP8232 -vascular adhesion protein-1 inhibitors).
- Insulin-like growth factor (IGF-1) inhibitors.
- Teprotumumab (RV001) is an IGF-1 inhibitor (intravenous infusion).
- TIME-2 study – AKB-9778 Tie2 activator, stabilizes blood vessels, prevents angiogenesis, and reduces vascular permeability. When combined with RBZ, it decreases DME better in comparison to anti-VEGF alone.

New Agents (Some are for AMD, but may have applications in vascular diseases)

Abicipar pegol (Allergan) – SEQUOIA, CEDAR, MAPLE trials in n-AMD; high rates of inflammation and vasculitis haemorrhagic.	**AKB-9778 (Aerpio Pharmaceutical)** – TIME trial in severe NPDR. Subcutaneous injection – inhibits tryrosine phosphatase – regulates Tie2 – improves DR and RFT.	**THR-317 (Oxurion)** – anti placental growth factor antibody in DME, JFMT-1, **THR-149** – plasma Kallikren inhibitor and **THR-687** – an integrin antagonist.
DE-122 (Carotuximab, Santen) – antibody to endoglin (angiogenic protein) expressed by endothelium and upregulated by anti-VEGF for refractory nAMD.	**Risuteganib (Luminate, Allergo Ophthalmics)** – anti-Integrin peptide, in DME and dry AMD. Targets four oxidative stress pathways – vascular permeability, angiogenesis, cell death, neurodegeneration. DELMAR trial.	**Farcimab (RG7716, Roche/Genentech)** – Anti-VEGF + anti Angiopoietin-2, bispecific antibody- in n-AMD, DME. Trials – STAIRWAY, YOSEMITE, RHINE.
		OPT-302 (Ophthea) – Trap mechanism, inhibits VEGF-C and D, in nAMD.
KSi-301 (Kodiak Science) – anti VEGF biopolymer conjugate in DME, RVO, and n-AMD.	**Valeda light delivery system (LumThera)** – reduces metabolic dysfunction, inflammation by photo-biomodulation in dry AMD LIGHTSITE trial.	**GB-102 (Graybug Vision)** – Sunitinib maleate-tyrosine kinase inhibitor, pan VEGFR antagonist, ADAGIO, PRELUDE trials.
AKST-4290 (Alkahest inc) – oral CCR3 inhibitor in nAMD.	**Elamipretide (Stealth Bio)** – subcutaneous injection in dry AMD, Leber's HON, mitochondrial myopathy.	**APL-2 (Apellis Pharmaceuticals)** (Apellis pharma) – DERBY, OAKS, FILLY trials – inhibitor of complement factor C3 for GA.

ICON-1 (Iconic therapeutics) – tissue factor antagonist, in wet AMD, EMERGE, DECO trials.
PAN-90806 (PanOptica) – topical selective anti-VEGFR, in nAMD, DME, RVO.
Zimura (Ophthotech corp) – Avacincaptag pegol, complement factor C5 inhibitor.

Port delivery system with Ranibizumab (Roche/Genentec) – **PDS** Refillable eye implant, for nAMD, Ladder, Archway trials. Implant is surgically placed in pars plana, to provide slow continuous release of RBZ for 6 months, between refills.

5.2 APPROACH TO DIABETIC EYE DISEASE

The prevalence of diabetes is increasing due to industrialization and changing lifestyles, and projected to rise to 370 million in 2030. Diabetic retinopathy is a leading cause of preventable visual loss in the working-age population of developed countries. DR usually develops after 14–15 years of mediocre diabetic control. With good control, this can be delayed for longer.

The DCCT trial (diabetes control and complication trial) and UK prospective diabetic study confirmed that improved control of BSL, BP, and serum lipids reduced the incidence and severity of retinopathy in diabetic patients. **Every 1% reduction in HbA1C caused a 35% reduction in onset and progression of retinopathy**.

Risk factors for diabetic retinopathy/maculopathy include:

- Duration, age, genetic predisposition, and ethnicity (**non-modifiable risk factors**).

- Longer duration, poor control, sudden changes in BSL (improvement/worsening), starting/changing insulin, frequent hyper/hypoglycaemia, and HbA1c < 3% (9 mmol/mol) cause progression of DR.

- Pregnancy.

- Cardiovascular problems, hypertension, anaemia, and sleep apnoea, worsen retinal hypoxia (ACE inhibitors are protective in DME).

- **DR risk increases by 35% for every 1% HbA1c rise, 1.1% for every 1 mm systolic BP >115 mmHg; and smoking each cigarette causes a 20% increase**. These are **modifiable risk factors**.

- Nephropathy, causing intravascular fluid overload and hypoalbuminemia, has a strong association with severe DR.

- Hyperlipidaemia causes severe and persistent exudative maculopathy (important to treat with statins, fibrates, and ACE inhibitors).

- Obesity is associated with poor diabetic control and insulin resistance.

- Smoking worsens exudation and cardiovascular risks.

- Cataract surgery leads to worsening of DR, due to inflammatory stimulus.

- **Rosiglitazone and pioglitazone** should not be used in the presence of significant retinopathy and maculopathy, as they increase macular oedema and fluid retention.

5.2.1 Pathogenesis of Diabetic Retinopathy

DR is a microvascular angiopathy (disease of retinal capillaries), compromising vascular integrity due to prolonged hyperglycaemia with associated inflammatory changes. Weakness of capillary walls causes microaneurysm and loss of pericytes results in leaky tight junctions, causing exudation and oedema. DME results from disruption of the blood-retinal barrier and imbalance of vascular hydrostatic and tissue oncotic pressure, driven by Starling's law.

Endothelial cell proliferation, and alteration of capillary basement membrane thickness, impairs diffusion and transfer of oxygen, nutrients, and metabolites leading to stasis, ischaemia, and hypoxic injury from capillary shutdown. This is clinically evident by the presence of CWS, IRMAs, neovascularization, and areas of capillary nonperfusion on FFA. Choroidal ischaemia worsens the condition by affecting RPE function. VEGF, inflammatory cytokines, and growth factors (PDGF, HGF, interleukins, TNF-a) released by the ischaemic retina play a crucial role in disease development.

5.2.2 ETDRS Classification and Clinical Signs of DR

The Early Treatment Diabetic Retinopathy Study classification, used internationally, classifies DR as non-proliferative DR (NPDR – mild, moderate, and severe) or proliferative DR (PDR).

The incidence of NPDR is 25% at 5 years, rising to 80% at 15 years from time of diagnosis. The incidence of PDR is 2% at 5 years, rising to 15.5 % at 15 years.

Mild NPDR – FU yearly interval by DRSS.
Microaneurysms (mA) – earliest detectable sign, seen as small (15–100 µm), well-defined red dots, **more visible with red-free and FFA images**.
Retinal haemorrhages – occur when mA rupture. Size >125 µm.
Superficial Hx are flame shaped, in the nerve fibre layer.
Deep Hx are dot and blot shaped, in the outer plexiform/inner nuclear layer.

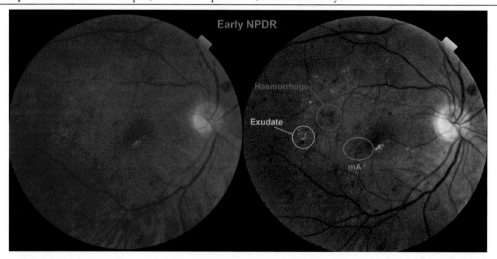

Figure 5.1 Early NPDR.

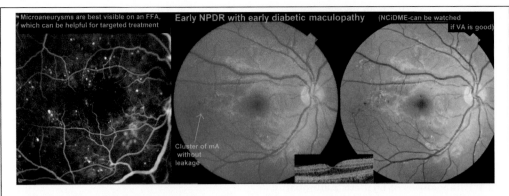

Figure 5.2 Moderately Severe NPDR – 1.

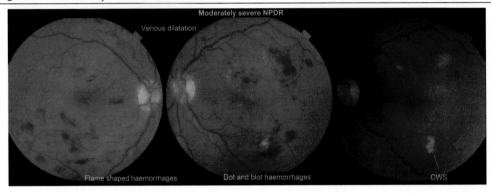

Figure 5.3 Moderately Severe NPDR – 2.

Moderate NPDR – FU at 4–6 monthly intervals in the eye clinic.
- **Hard exudates** – active or resolved leakage from altered vascular permeability, leaves whitish-yellow cholesterol and lipoprotein deposits in the outer plexiform layer, more common at the macula, and can affect vision with foveal involvement.
- **Cotton-wool spots or soft exudates** – are fluffy, feathery white areas of RNFL infarction, generally at the posterior pole (RNFL is thickest), and spontaneously clear in a few weeks. Presence of multiple infarcts is suggestive of ischaemia.
- **Venous beading and looping** – representing weakened walls of major retinal vessels, with saccular bulges, often adjacent to areas of non-perfusion. **It is one of the strongest predictors for progression to proliferative diabetic retinopathy,** with a 12–27% risk of developing PDR within 1 year.

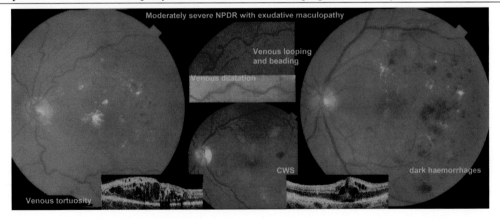

Figure 5.4 Moderately severe NPDR with exudative maculopathy.

Severe NPDR (pre-proliferative DR) – needs active FU at 3–4 monthly intervals, consider prophylactic PRP in high-risk patients.
- **4-2-1 rule** – >20 intraretinal haemorrhages in **4 quadrants** + venous beading in **2 or more quadrants** + IRMA in **1 or more quadrants**.
- **Intraretinal microvascular abnormality (IRMA)** – small abnormal vessels that shunt blood from arterioles to venules. They appear adjacent to nonperfused areas, and do not leak on FFA. **IRMA are precursors to NVE and need close monitoring.**
- Patients with severe NPDR have **more than 50% risk of developing PDR within 1 year, high risk of neuropathy and permanent visual loss.**

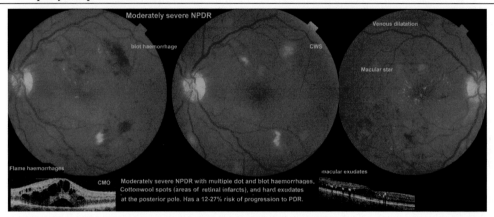

Figure 5.5 Severe NPDR to PDR.

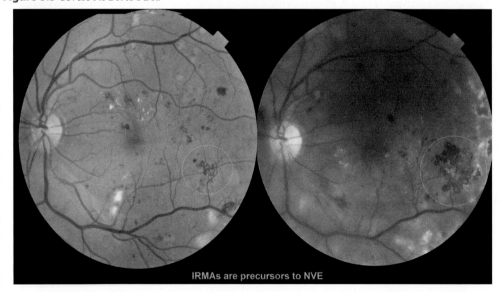

Figure 5.6 IRMA to NVE.

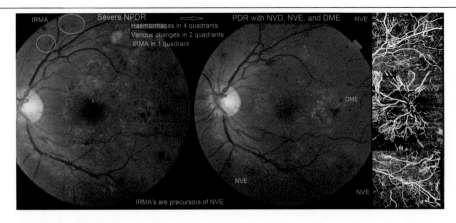

Figure 5.7 Severe NPDR.

Proliferative DR (PDR) – needs urgent treatment with laser photocoagulation.
The main stimulus for neovascularization is retinal hypoxia (manifest by capillary dropout on FFA),
endothelial cell disruption, and production of angiogenic growth factors. Retinal non-perfusion >25% leads
to development of PDR.
- **Neovascularization** – development of NVD (NV on disc/within 1DD of disc), NVE (NV anywhere on the
  retina 1DD away from the disc), NVA and NVI (NVG)
- **Vitreous haemorrhage, preretinal haemorrhage** – bleed from NVD/NVE.
- **Preretinal haemorrhage** – blood trapped in potential space between posterior hyaloid and ILM, appears as
  boat-shaped bleed.
- **Vitreous haemorrhage** – blood in vitreous cavity, affecting fundal view. Over time, the blood becomes de-
  haemoglobinized, and eventually turns white.

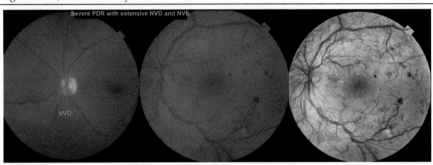

Figure 5.8 Severe PDR.

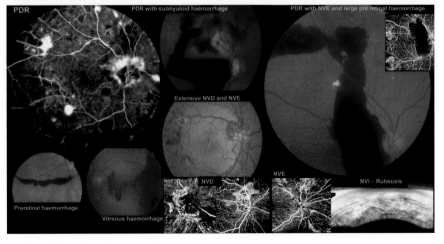

Figure 5.9 Montage of PDR.

- New vessels are sight-threatening because they are fragile, tend to bleed, and cause fibrosis and membrane formation. They are hyperfluorescent vessels with active leakage on FFA, and easy to identify on OCT-A.
- PDR are classified as low-risk or high-risk PDR, based on the DRS study. Eyes with high-risk PDR have severe vision loss (25–37% in 2 years) without treatment. High-risk criteria include:
  - NVD of more than quarter to one third of disc area.
  - Any NVD with vitreous haemorrhage.
  - NVE of more than ½ disc area with vitreous haemorrhage.
  - NVI or NVA.

End stage DR – associated with aggressive, active PDR, extensive PRP, and poor prognosis.
- **Tractional retinal detachment (TRD).**
- **Extensive fibrosis with retinal or macular distortion, heavy PRP scars.**
- **Rubeotic glaucoma.**

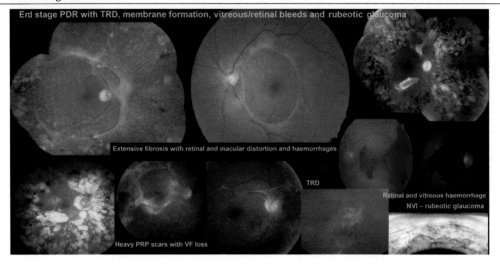

Figure 5.10 Montage of end-stage PDR.

Diabetic maculopathy – classified as:
- **Non-ischaemic maculopathy** – can be exudative, serous (oedema), or mixed. Usually, presents with good VA and good macular perfusion.
  - **Exudative maculopathy – presents with hard exudates (HE),** which can be focal or circinate in distribution.
  - **Macular star** – lipid accumulates in the layer of Henle surrounding the macula.
  - **Macular oedema (DME)** – intraretinal or subretinal fluid collection.
- **Ischaemic maculopathy** – poor vision with subtle changes, featureless macula with persistent oedema, enlarged FAZ on FFA and OCT-A, worse visual prognosis.
- **Mixed maculopathy** – elements of exudative + ischaemic maculopathy

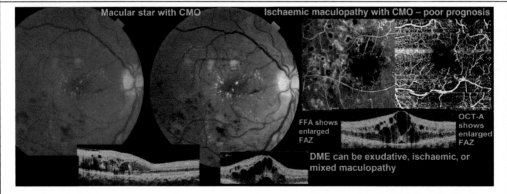

Figure 5.11 Diabetic maculopathy.

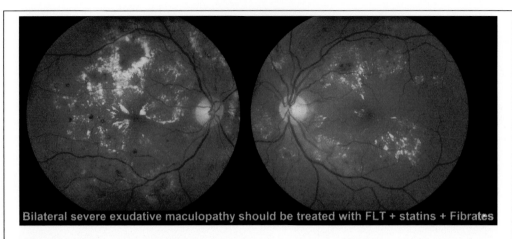

Bilateral severe exudative maculopathy should be treated with FLT + statins + Fibrates

Figure 5.12 Bilateral severe exudative maculopathy.

Diabetic Macular Oedema
DME is accumulation of fluid between the outer plexiform and inner nuclear layers, associated with swelling of Müller cells, and expansion of intra and extracellular spaces in the macular area, secondary to abnormal permeability of the perimacular capillaries (failure of inner blood-retinal barrier) and RPE (outer retinal barrier). This leads to accumulation of interstitial fluid, representing the most important reason for visual loss in diabetic patients, with more than 50% of untreated patients losing more than 2 lines within 2 years. Photoreceptor layer atrophy is the most likely cause of visual loss.
CSME ETDRS criteria (clinically significant macular oedema):
• Retinal thickening within 500 μm of fovea.
• Hard exudates within 500 μm of fovea with associated retinal thickening.
• Retina thickening >1 disc area (1500 μm) located within 1 disc diameter of the fovea.

In the **OCT era**, ETDRS criteria are no longer relevant. OCT can better visualize and quantify macular oedema. We now talk of **centre involving DME (CiDME)** or **non-centre involving DME (NCiDME)**

• **FFA and OCT are essential tools in assessment and management of DME. OCT-A has the potential to replace FFA in the future.**

• FFA shows site of leakage, extent of ischaemia (retinal/macular), and early NV.
• OCT determines the extent and type of retinal thickening, presence of structural changes, and response to treatment.
• Documentation of DME should include the following criteria, which decide treatment protocols and predicts prognosis:

Location on macular map central/nasal/temporal	Type – diffuse/focal cystoid/SRF/IRF	+/− VMT, ERM, submacular fibrosis
Amount: thickness – CRT	+/− chronic	+/− exudates

• **Worse prognostic features include** – presence of submacular exudates, IRC, SRF, chronicity, sub-foveal fibrosis, structural changes (scarring, RPE atrophy, ERM, VMT, and macular holes), and macular ischaemia.

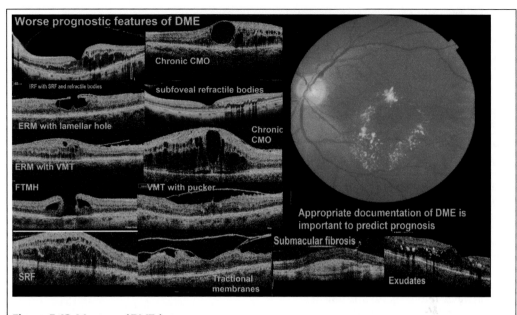

Figure 5.13 Montage of DME features.

Diabetic maculopathy can be classified by presentation, location, and appearance.

DME Categorized by Clinical or OCT Presentation
- **Focal DME** (localized leakage from microaneurysms) or **diffuse DME** – oedema involves entire area on the macular map.
- **Cystoid DME** – intra-retinal cystic fluid **or serous detachment** – sub-retinal fluid.

DME Categorized by Location
- **Centre-involving DME and non-centre involving DME.**

DME Classified on Appearance
- **Exudative maculopathy** – cluster of microaneurysms associated with exudates and circinate. Good prognosis with laser treatment.
- **Ischaemic maculopathy** – oedema associated with poor macular perfusion. Poor prognosis with laser treatment, IVT preferred.
- **Mixed maculopathy** – combination of exudative + ischaemic maculopathy.

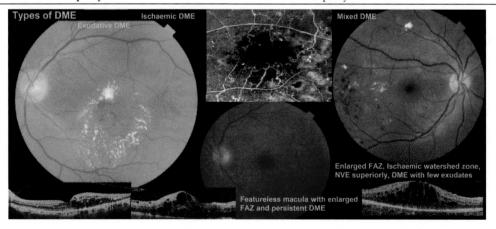

Figure 5.14 Types of DME.

5.2.3 Management of Diabetic Retinopathy

The diabetic retinopathy screening service, using high-quality fundal imaging, has improved diagnosis, referral, and routine monitoring of diabetic eye disease in the community.

181

Normal levels recommended by the American Diabetic Association			
Parameters	Target values	Parameters	Target values
BP HbA1C Fasting BSL Postprandial BSL	<130 / 80mm of Hg <7% (50mmol/mol) 90 -130mg/dl <180mg/dl	Triglycerides LDL HDL RFT	< 150mg/dl < 100mg/dl > 40mg/dl < 30um/mg creatinine
Early treatment of all risk factors is associated with better prognosis.			

Figure 5.15 Normal blood levels in DM.

Current treatment strategy is to prevent any further visual loss.

Significant visual loss is related to DME and vitreous haemorrhage. Other causes include refractive fluctuations, cataracts, development of structural changes like VMT, ERM, macular pucker, atrophy, haemorrhage, or laser burns and scars.

Vision rarely improves after treatment, and the best results are achieved with early treatment. Central vision can remain surprisingly good despite marked capillary closure, provided treatment is done before foveal involvement. With mixed maculopathy, prognosis depends on the extent and location of oedema and severity of ischaemia.

Ischaemic maculopathy is common in older diabetics with poor control and co-existing cardio-vascular conditions. Visual loss from macular ischaemia does not improve with FLT, and laser can worsen the vision.

Laser treatment remains the gold standard for diabetic retinopathy and non-centre involving maculopathy.

IVT – anti-VEGF and steroids offer better visual outcomes with CiDME but are offset by the ongoing nature of treatment, with associated socio-economic costs, that far exceed costs of laser treatment.

A **combination therapy** – anti-VEGF injections, followed by laser treatment – may help maintain vision and stabilize disease.

The mainstay treatments are:

- **Anti-VEGF for DME.**

- **PRP for high-risk PDR.**

- **Surgery (vitrectomy) for non-clearing vitreous haemorrhage or TRDs.**

Newer lasers (micro-pulse, subthreshold, and longer wavelengths) offer substantial improvement in treatment and outcomes. They reduce retinal damage and lead to retinal rejuvenation and visual improvement, renewing interest in laser therapy, due to the increasing work burden and spiralling costs associated with IVT.

5.2.4 Treatment Strategies

Clinical trials and landmark studies provide evidence for effective treatment strategies, based on disease presentation, severity, treatment availability, compliance, co-morbidity, costs, and socio-economic issues.

Retinal photocoagulation, either alone or combined with pharmacological therapy, remains the standard of care for diabetic retinal disease.

Common lasers in use are:

- Argon green (514.4 nm).

- PASCAL (532 nm – green, yellow – 577 nm).

- Micro-pulse diode laser (810 nm – red).

Several RCTs, prove the efficacy of treatment in diabetic eye disease.

The Wisconsin Epidemiological Study of DR (WESDR) – linked severity of DR/DME to duration of diabetes.
The Diabetes Control and Complication Trial (DCCT) – found DME in T2DM > T1DM.
The Diabetic Retinopathy Study (DRS) – reported 10% visual loss after PRP in PDR, but 25–40% with co-existing DME. So, PDR without DME tolerates PRP well.
The Early Treatment Diabetic Retinopathy Study (ETDRS) – found that early PRP reduced severe visual loss by >50% and FLT reduced moderate visual loss from DME by 50% in 3 years.
The Ranibizumab for oEdema of the mAcula in Diabetes-2 (READ-2) – demonstrated that RBZ was better than laser, but combination therapy may reduce injection frequency.
Several RCTs – **RESOLVE, VIVID/VISTA, RISE/RIDE, DRCR.net, RESTORE, REVEAL and Da-Vinci study** – have confirmed the beneficial effects of IVT in DME. **IVT with anti-VEGF is standard treatment for CiDME with CRT >400 μm.**

The Diabetic Retinopathy Clinical Research Network (DRCR.net)
- **Protocol A** – demonstrated efficacy of modified grid laser for DME.
- **Protocol B** – FLT vs IVTA for DME. Laser more effective, fewer side-effects.
- **Protocol I** – RBZ + prompt or deferred (>24 wks) FLT vs IVTA or sham + prompt laser. RBZ + laser arm more effective than steroid or sham arms.
- **Protocol S** – IV ranibizumab monotherapy was as effective as PRP in PDR.
- **Protocol T** – compared all three anti-VEGF agents in DME. All equally effective in DME with good vision. **When baseline vision was 20/50 or worse, aflibercept had a better initial visual and anatomical outcome (not sustained at 2 years).**
- **Protocol U** – compared IV Ranibizumab vs RBZ + Dexa-implant (Ozurdex) for persistent DME. No added benefit of combination therapy.
- **Protocol V** – evaluated CiDME with good vision (>20/25), and found no significant loss at 2 years with IV aflibercept vs laser vs observation. So patients with good vision can be safely monitored, and only treated if vision worsens.

Other Studies
Panorama study – benefit of aflibercept in severe NPDR.
Fame study – benefit of fenofibrate in T1DM.
The Ozurdex PLACID, MEAD, Bevordex, Famous and Champlain study – evaluated benefits and side-effects of the Dexa implant in diffuse DME.
The Diabetic Retinopathy Vitrectomy Study – explored benefits of early vitrectomy.

Regression rates are 75%, 67%, and 43% for mild, moderate, and severe PDR, following PRP. A complete PRP reduces VF by 40–50%, but this can be limited to 20% by using small spots, low energy, and large gaps.

Type 1 diabetics should have annual screenings for DR, 5 years after onset of disease, while type 2 diabetics should have prompt screening at diagnosis and yearly thereafter. Maintaining good BSL and BP lowers risk of development or progression of retinopathy. Diabetics have accelerated progression during puberty and pregnancy and should be closely monitored.

Monitoring for disease progression and treatment response is done using objective metrics – fundal photography, OCT, OCT-A, FFA, and perimetry. Recent advances in Big Data, machine-learning algorithms, and artificial intelligence can be applied to diabetic eye disease, to develop predictive models and risk calculators based on all risk factors, for better prediction, early detection, and treatment of DR.

Current models, based on screening all diabetics to identify the few (10% with VTDR – visually threatening DR) that require active treatment, are expensive and labour intensive. AI stratifies risks accurately, predicting disease development in advance, allowing early detection and treatment of modifiable risk factors, to prevent development or worsening of DR. Targeted treatment, in a timely fashion, reduces overall cost to the healthcare system and improves prognosis.

Diabetic Retinopathy Treatment – Ready Reckoner	
No DR Mild DR	First review 3–5 years after diagnosis. Yearly FU with screening service. Advice on control of all modifiable risk factors for DR.
Moderate NPDR	Observation + improve BSL, clinic review at 6/12 intervals.
Severe NPDR	Close observation at 3/12 interval **PRP in high risk patients – 2000–3000 burns in 2 sessions** (poor attenders, nephropathy, only eye, pregnancy, PDR-other eye).
Low-risk PDR	**Urgent PRP** – 2–3 sessions at 3–4 wks × 1000–1500 burns/visit. **Total of 2500–4500 burns.** Review in 2/12. Top up if active.
High-risk PDR Multiple, forward-growing NV	**Urgent PRP – 4–5 sessions fractionated PRP** at shorter intervals (4–7 days) × 800–1000 burns/session – to reduce risks and complications of excessive fibrosis. **Total of 4000–6000 burns**, review in 2/12. Top up if active.

Iris neovascularization	NVI or NVA without retinal NV – needs aggressive treatment. **Urgent PRP** – 2–3 sessions× 1500–2500 burns/session at short intervals. **Total of 4000–6000 burns** within 2–3 weeks. Review in a few weeks for IOP check, top up if still active.
Vitreous haemorrhage	Await clearance, then PRP based on activity. If limited retinal view available – start PRP (aids clearance). Young patients with active PDR, consider IV Avastin, aids clearance, and allow PRP.
PRP may worsen DME. Treat DME 4–6 weeks prior to PRP or consider IVT if urgent PRP required. PRP at 4–6 week intervals and in the far periphery reduces risk of DME.	
VR referral – for pars plana vitrectomy, endo-laser, removal of fibrovascular bands, IVT, membrane peel, and TPA +gas. • Persistent vitreous haemorrhage >2/12. • Extensive PDR, poor response to PRP. • Active DR/extensive PRP – no more room. • TRD, extensive fibrovascular band, macular or retinal distortion. • ERM, macular pucker, hole. • Sub-macular haemorrhage. • VMT with persistent/recalcitrant MO (33%).	**Medical treatment** • Improve BSL, BP, blood lipids – reduces haemorrhages, leakage and exudation. • Stop smoking (×4 risk of DR). • Consider ACE inhibitors. • Fibrates and statins. • Avoid Rosiglitazone and Pioglitazone. • Weight loss. • Stable RFT.
Diabetic maculopathy – early treatment before fovea involvement leads to better outcomes.	
No DME	Observation – screening services
Non CiDME	FLT, Modified grid laser. Review in 4/12 + OCT scan.
CiDME, CRT <400 µm	VA >20/25 – observe or FLT in phakic patients. IVTA in pseudophakes
CRT >400 µm	IV anti VEGF (RBZ, BVZ or AFL). Aflibercept ×5 loading dose is preferred over other IVT, especially in chronic cases. Steroid implants may be considered, in pseudophakes. Grid laser treatment if patient refuses IVT. Partial response or persistent exudates – add deferred FLT.
Persistent/non-responsive DME (no improvement after 3 IVT or FLT).	Repeat FFA – targeted FLT. Review 4/12. Reload anti-VEGF, switch to aflibercept, switch to steroids. Combination therapy – target different pathways and action duration. Anti-VEGF (immediate) + steroids/FLT (long term).
Ischaemic DME	IV aflibercept preferred (protocol V), guarded prognosis. Avoid further laser. May have retinal ischaemia – needing PRP.
Pregnancy + DME (15–25%) – DIEP study	Observation, improve BSL, FLT, IV steroids in 2nd and 3rd trimester in refractory cases. Avoid anti-VEGF (no safety data).

5.3 APPROACH TO RETINAL VEIN OCCLUSION

Retinal vein occlusions are the second most common retinal vascular disease after diabetic retinopathy, and can affect a branch vein (BRVO), hemi-vein (HRVO), or the central retinal vein (CRVO). BRVOs are six times more common than CRVO, with no significant difference across race, gender, and ethnicity. Although RVOs are common in the sixth/seventh decade, 49% of patients are younger than 65, with 15% CRVO, 10% HRVO, and 5% BRVO patients younger than 45 years.

An RVO can be complete or partial, with increased intravenous pressure, causing proximal venous dilatation, intraretinal haemorrhages, and leakage.

CRVO and HRVOs present with acute painless visual loss and have similar clinical course and pathophysiology. Visual loss is due to macular oedema, intra-retinal haemorrhage, macular, or neovascularization causing vitreous bleed. The prognosis varies based on site and type of occlusion (ischaemic or non-ischaemic). In general, a more-distal, non-ischaemic occlusion has a better prognosis than a proximal, ischaemic blockage. Occasionally, an RVO may occur concurrently with a retinal artery occlusion.

5.3.1 Risk Factors for RVO

Age and systemic vascular diseases are strongly associated with RVO, confirmed by DCCT and Blue Mountain studies.

The triad of HT, DM, and hyperlipidaemia is commonly present in 25–30% of CRVO and 35–40% of BRVO cases and its presence increases the risk of developing RVO by 58%.

• **Age – commonest in 6th and 8th decade** • **Men slightly higher risk than women** • **Lower socio-economic group** • **Drugs** – OC pills, diuretics, hypotensive agents	• **Smoking** • **Obesity and associated problems** – sleep apnoea • Family history
• **Systemic cardio-vascular factors** – hypertension (48% risk), hyperlipidaemia (20%), coronary artery disease, carotid occlusive disease, atherosclerosis, myocardial infarction, deep vein thrombosis (DVT), peripheral vascular disease, and pulmonary embolism. The risk increases with severity of systemic disease.	
• **Metabolic disease** – diabetes mellitus (5% risk), obesity (high body-mass index), and vitamin B6 and folic acid deficiency.	
• **Hypercoagulable state – all causes of increased plasma viscosity** – leukaemia, lymphoma, polycythaemia vera, thrombocythemia, sickle cell disease, multiple myeloma, malignancies, pregnancy.	
• **Inflammatory diseases** – SLE, sarcoidosis, syphilis, Bechet's syndrome, vasculitis.	
• **Thrombophilia (important in young patients with RVO)** – elevated homocysteine level, factor V Leiden, anti-phospholipid syndrome, protein C and S deficiency, anti-cardiolipin antibodies.	
RVOs are less common in patients under 40, with unusual presentations, more proximal blockage, bilateral involvement, and personal or family history of thrombosis. They are associated with hypercoagulability, vasculitis, and congenital thrombophilia.	
• **Ocular factors – risk for BRVO.** • Local vascular changes (ocular) – AV crossing changes, superior quadrant. • Retinal phlebitis, glaucoma, and OHT. • External retrobulbar compression – tumour, endocrine orbitopathy.	

A previous history of RVO in one eye is a risk factor (10% over 3 years) for an RVO in the fellow eye. Smoking and systemic inflammatory and vascular conditions increase this risk. Optimizing control of risk factors, especially the triad of hypertension, diabetes, and hyperlipidaemia, and improving IOP control, are important in management of RVO.

5.3.2 Pathogenesis of RVO

The pathogenesis is not completely understood but involves a triad of vessel wall injury/degeneration, venous stasis, and blood coagulopathy, known as **Virchow's triad.**

The retinal venule occlusion is always secondary to atherosclerosis of adjacent

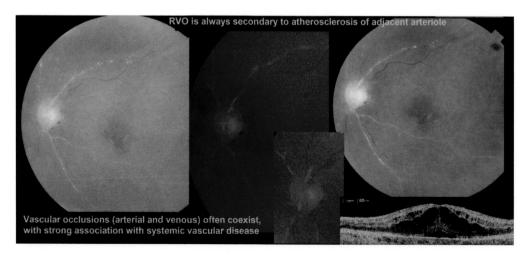

Figure 5.16 RVO + arterial disease.

arteriole, explaining the strong association with systemic vascular diseases.

5.3.3 Location of RVO

- **CRVO** – occlusion of main retinal vein at the optic disc.

- **Hemi-vein occlusion** – occlusion of superior or inferior hemi-vein.

- **Branch vein occlusion** – involves branch veins in the four quadrants (ST, SN, IT, IN), or macular branch vein.

CRVO and HRVO are proximal occlusions with similar pathophysiology, outcomes, and complications. They are associated with a high risk of anterior segment neovascularization (NVI and NVA) and neovascular glaucoma.

BRVO and HRVO commonly occur at a point of AV crossing, and can be associated with CMO, exudates, epiretinal membrane, RAM, CRAO, or cilioretinal artery occlusion.

5.3.3.1 Type of Retinal Venous Occlusion

RVOs are classified into **ischaemic** and **non-ischaemic** based on degree of capillary non-perfusion seen on FFA. *(Extent of ischaemia determined by CVOS study, defined an ischaemic CRVO as at least 10-disc areas of capillary non-perfusion).*

Differentiating subtypes is important because it predicts natural progression of RVO, response to treatment, outcomes, and visual prognosis. However, **it is now known that all RVOs are ischaemic to some degree, and the spectrum of capillary nonperfusion can vary and progress.**

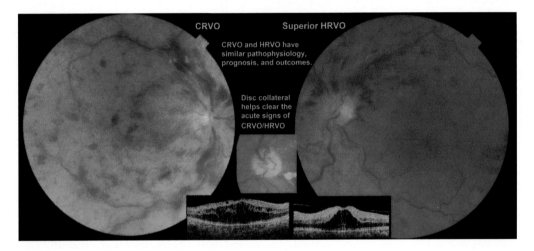

Figure 5.17 CRVO and HRVO.

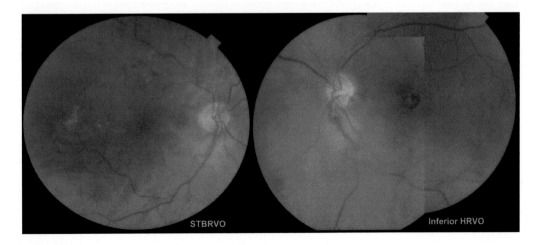

Figure 5.18 BRVO and HRVO.

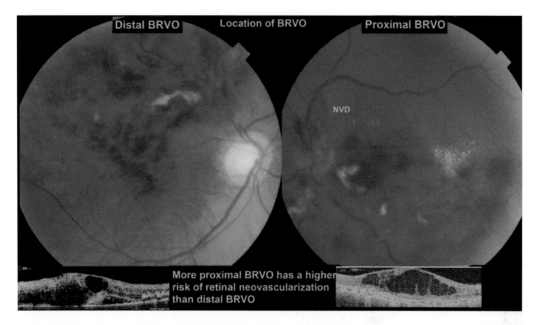

Figure 5.19 Distal vs proximal BRVO.

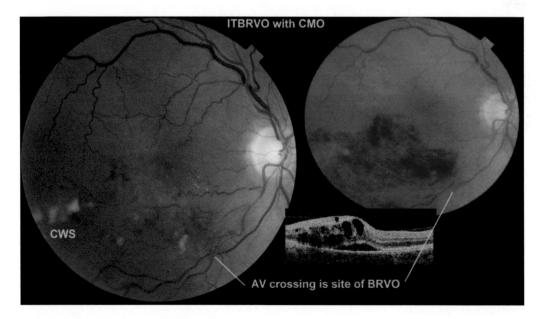

Figure 5.20 ITBRVO – site of blockage.

As the affected retina releases hypoxic factors like VEGF, a non-ischaemic RVO can convert to an ischaemic RVO with time.

Approximately 70–80% of CRVO are non-ischaemic and resolve spontaneously with good anatomical and visual outcomes. A few cases progress to the ischaemic type, developing neovascularization and neovascular glaucoma (60–70% risk with ischaemic CRVO). It is important to identify this cohort to plan early treatment and prevent these complications. Ischaemic CRVO (20%) are associated with worse VA on presentation and poor visual prognosis despite treatment.

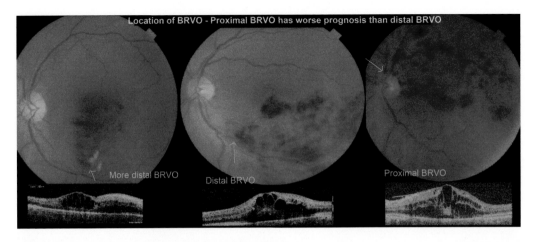

Figure 5.21 Location of BRVO.

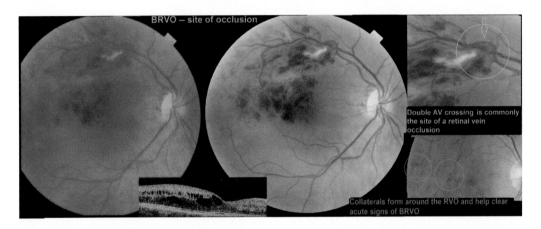

Figure 5.22 BRVO with site of occlusion.

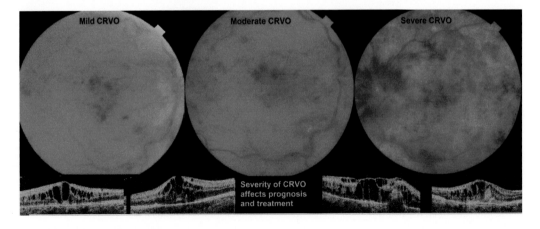

Figure 5.23 Severity of CRVO.

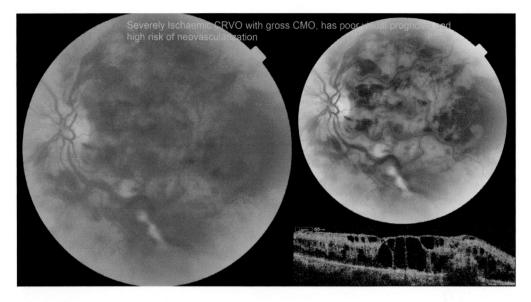

Figure 5.24 Severely ischaemic CRVO with high risk of NV.

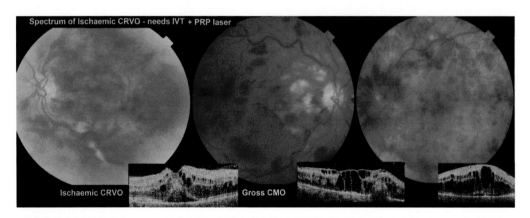

Figure 5.25 Spectrum of Ischaemic CRVO.

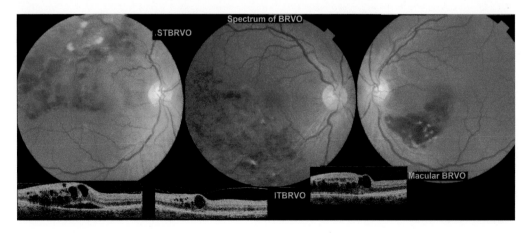

Figure 5.26 spectrum of BRVO.

5.3.3.2 How Do You Assess Extent of Ischaemia?

Retinal ischaemia is traditionally assessed using FFA. *(The Central Retinal Vein Occlusion Study (CVOS) defined ischaemia, as ≥10 disc diameters of non-perfusion on FFA).* Accurately assessing the full extent of retinal ischaemia can be challenging.

The predictive value of FFA can be unreliable due to assessment variability and difficulties in defining ischaemic areas, masked by media opacities or haemorrhages in the acute phase. Additionally, documentation is not standardized, and ischaemia may progress for up to 3 months following CRVO. A standard seven-field FFA view only captures one third of the retina, missing significant amounts of peripheral ischaemia. **An FFA may therefore underestimate the extent of retinal ischaemia.** Wide field imaging technology has improved assessment and should be used if available. CVOS showed 16% of patients developed rubeosis, of which 48% were initially classified as perfused on FFA.

Functional visual tests are deemed better at assessing ischaemia, including visual acuity, visual field, relative afferent pupillary defect, and ERG. Ideally, a combination of functional tests, clinical examination, FFA, and UWFA are used to assess ischaemia.

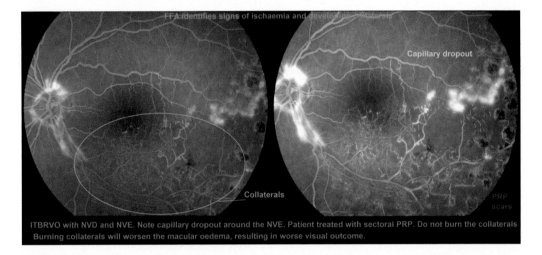

ITBRVO with NVD and NVE. Note capillary dropout around the NVE. Patient treated with sectoral PRP. Do not burn the collaterals Burning collaterals will worsen the macular oedema, resulting in worse visual outcome.

Figure 5.27 FFA in ITBRVO.

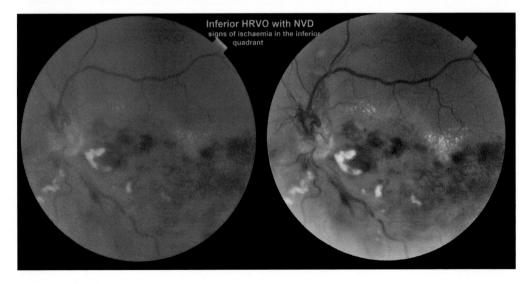

Figure 5.28 HRVO with NVD.

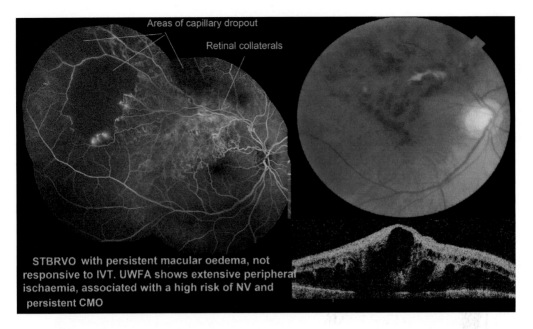

Areas of capillary dropout

Retinal collaterals

STBRVO with persistent macular oedema, not responsive to IVT. UWFA shows extensive peripheral ischaemia, associated with a high risk of NV and persistent CMO

Figure 5.29 STBRVO with peripheral ischaemia.

Several studies have confirmed that 30 Hz photopic flicker ERG is quick and superior to FFA in predicting rubeosis development. Reduced a-wave, increased b-wave amplitude, reversed b:a ratio, and prolonged b-wave implicit time indicate retinal ischaemia on ERG.

Hayreh et al. identified high-risk characteristics in CRVO patients, including BCVA (best corrected visual acuity) ≤ 6/60, loss of 1–2e isopter on Goldmann visual field, RAPD ≥0.9 log units determined by neutral density filters, and ERG reduction ≤60% of a-wave.

5.3.3.3 Clinical Features of Ischaemic Retinal Vein Occlusion

Although ERG, FFA, and VF predict the extent of ischaemia they are time-consuming and not always available in clinic. Urgent PRP is indicated for retinal or anterior segment neovascularization. Although prophylactic PRP is not recommended, clinicians must have a high index of suspicion and watch high-risk patients closely, involving frequent follow-up visits with a multitude of tests, making it less cost-effective. In a real-world scenario, if a patient is judged severely ischaemic, clinically or with tests, it is reasonable to consider early PRP.

Clinical features of severe ischaemia in CRVO and HRVO patients are:

Non-ischaemic CRVO	Ischaemic CRVO
VA – better than 6/60.	**VA worse than 6/60.**
	Strong association with cardiovascular problems.
Fewer haemorrhages. Few/No CWS.	Extensive haemorrhages, retinal oedema. Lots of CWS.
Less vascular tortuosity.	Very dilated, tortuous veins.
No/less disc swelling. No RAPD.	Disc swelling. **RAPD.**
FFA – good retinal perfusion, slight delay in AV transit time, leakage with CMO. Risk of NV is low.	FFA shows marked capillary non-perfusion. 60% risk of neovascularization within 3/12. Significant peripheral ischaemia present.
ERG – normal a-wave amplitude as inner retina is well perfused.	ERG shows > 60% reduced A-wave amplitude and b/a >1 – good predictor of ischaemia.
Goldmann VF – no peripheral VF loss.	Goldmann VF – loss of peripheral VF seen.

These patients were highly likely to develop rubeosis within 3 months (described as the 90-day glaucoma). The advent of IVT has reduced the VEGF drive, delaying onset of rubeosis, which typically manifests when the treatment is extended or delayed.

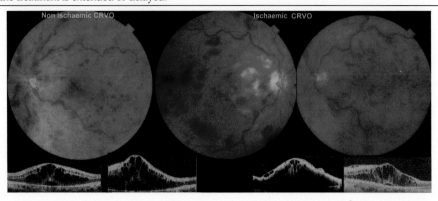

Figure 5.30 Ischaemic vs nonischaemic CRVO.

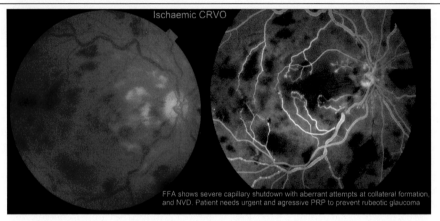

Figure 5.31 Ischaemic CRVO.

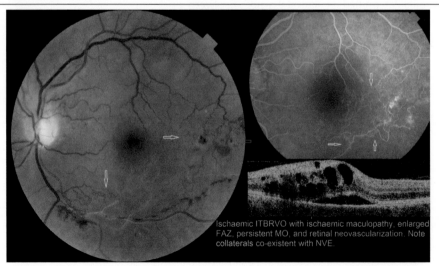

Figure 5.32 Ischaemic ITBRVO with NVE.

5.3.3.4 Ischaemia Associated with BRVO

Prognosis in BRVO depends on the degree of nonperfusion and location of occlusion. BRVO with severe non-perfusion can develop retinal NV and vitreous bleeds. There is a lower risk of anterior segment neovascularization.

Temporal BRVO can cause macular oedema in 30% of cases, with visual loss, distortion,

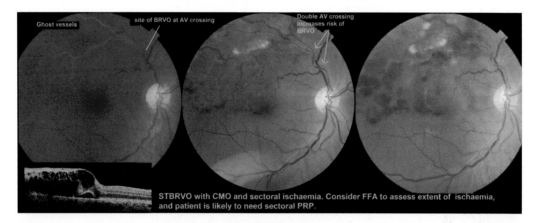

Figure 5.33 STBRVO with site of block and ghost vessels.

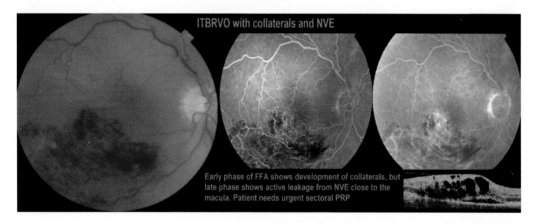

Figure 5.34 ITBRVO with collaterals and NVE.

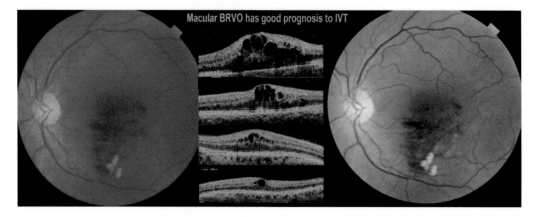

Figure 5.35 Macular BRVO has good prognosis.

and central scotoma. Nasal BRVO may go unrecognized and only be diagnosed on routine assessment or from a complication (vitreous bleed).

5.3.3.5 RVO Presentation

Early findings include vascular tortuosity, venous dilation, retinal oedema, intraretinal haemorrhages, cotton wool spots, hard exudates, and serous retinal detachment. The acute process resolves with clearance of haemorrhages but persistence of macular oedema, causing visual dysfunction. It may resolve over time, leaving secondary RPE atrophy, ERM, and suboptimal visual outcomes.

Collaterals develop between retinal venules and choroidal circulation at the disc following a CRVO and HRVO, and between the superior and inferior retinal veins in BRVO, usually at the junction of perfused and ischaemic retina. The development of collaterals helps venous drainage and resolution of macular oedema, and aids visual recovery. Collaterals represent healing blood vessels, and great care must be taken when lasering to avoid burning collaterals. **Damaging collaterals leads to worsening of macular oedema and visual outcomes.**

Collaterals may mimic new vessels but can be differentiated on an FFA. Unlike new vessels, collaterals are hyperfluorescent vessels that join up to surrounding vessels to bypass a blockage and do not leak on FFA. **Collaterals and new vessels may co-exist in an eye with RVO.**

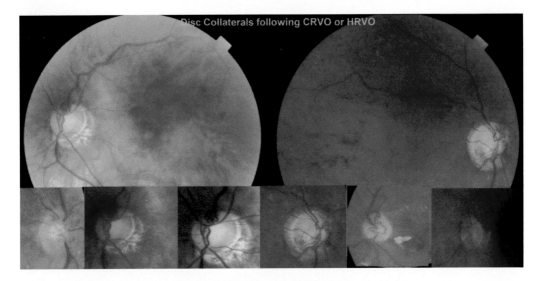

Figure 5.36 Disc collaterals following CRVO or HRVO.

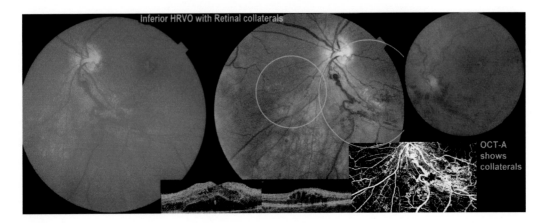

Figure 5.37 Inferior HRVO with collaterals.

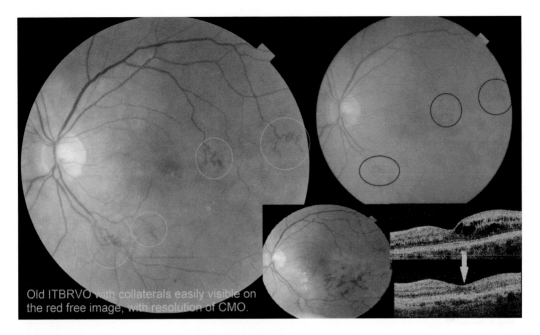

Figure 5.38 Non-ischaemic ITBRVO with good collaterals.

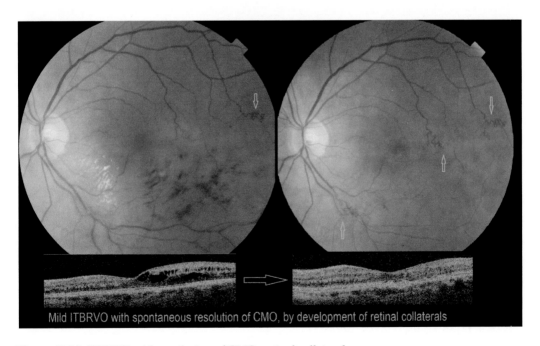

Figure 5.39 ITBRVO with resolution of CMO, retinal collateral.

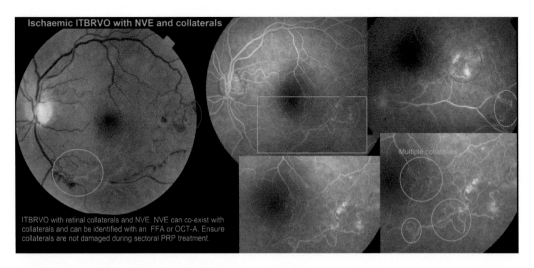

Figure 5.40 Ischaemic ITBRVO with NVE and collaterals.

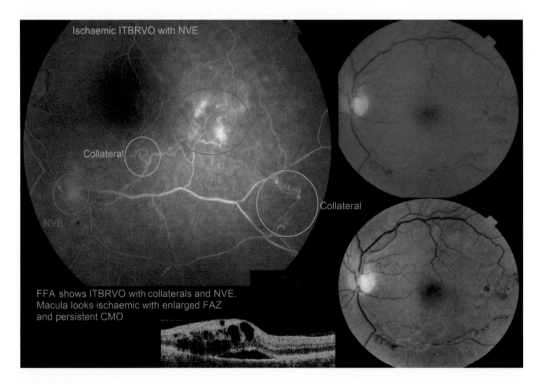

Figure 5.41 Ischaemic ITBRVO with NVE.

5.3.3.6 Assessment of RVO

Ocular Examination
<ul><li>VA (Snellen, logMAR), pupil reaction for RAPD, IOP to rule out glaucoma.</li><li>Gonioscopy – for NVA, a poorly dilated pupil may be the first indication of early NVI.</li><li>Fundoscopy – assess extent, location, and severity of RVO, presence of CMO and collaterals, and extent of peripheral ischaemia. **Clinical assessment is reasonably sensitive to determine the extent of ischaemia.**</li><li>Visual field test and ERG if available.</li></ul>

- **OCT** – to document and quantify CMO.
- **OCT-A** – helps detect capillary nonperfusion, enlarged FAZ, and neovascularization.
- **FFA** – evaluates extent of retinal and macular ischaemia and non-perfusion to guide effective laser treatment and distinguishes collateral from neovascularization. Haemorrhages mask fluorescence in the acute phase, limiting its value.
- **Ultra-wide field FFA** – detects peripheral ischaemia missed by standard FFA.

Systemic Work-up

- Cardiovascular work-up – BP, FBC, lipid profile, BSL.
- Extent of systemic evaluation is dependent on patient's age and medical history. Young patients with atypical presentation need investigation for systemic inflammatory conditions and inherited or acquired thrombophilia.
- **Inherited thrombophilia** – includes antithrombin deficiency, protein C and protein S, factor V Leiden, and the prothrombin G20210A mutation.
- **Acquired** risk factors for thrombosis include antiphospholipid antibody syndrome, myeloproliferative disorders, immobilization, major surgery, malignancy, oestrogen, and heparin-induced thrombocytopenia. Other risk factors include elevated levels of homocysteine and factors VIII, IX, and XI.

Studies in RVO

BRVO – BRAVO, HORIZON, RETAIN, SHORE, VIBRANT, SCORE, COBALT studies
CRVO – CRUISE, HORIZON, RETAIN, SHORE, COPERNICUS, GALILEO, GENEVA

SCORE study – macular grid laser recommended for well perfused BRVO with CMO.

VIBRANT study – laser vs aflibercept showed better outcomes with IVT.

CRUISE (CRVO) and **BRAVO** (BRVO) trials demonstrated efficacy of Ranibizumab.

SCORE2 study showed efficacy with bevacizumab or aflibercept in CRVO and HRVO.

Long-term studies (**HORIZON and RETAIN**) showed that visual gain was not always maintained beyond the first year with variability in response and recurrence rates.

Efficacy of intravitreal steroids (triamcinolone, dexamethasone, fluocinolone) were shown by **SCORE and GENEVA studies**. Steroids are reserved for pseudophakes, due to significant risk of development of cataracts and glaucoma.

BRIGHTER (2 years) and **RETAIN** (4 years) studies demonstrated that adding laser to ranibizumab did not result in a better visual outcome or reduce injection rates.

The **COPERNICUS study** (CRVO) showed no progression to neovascularization in the Aflibercept group compared to sham.

RELATE study – scatter PRP did not improve BCVA, reduce injections, or improve CMO. PRP is done to prevent neovascular complications, not for visual improvement.

RAVE (rubeosis anti-VEGF) trial in ischaemic CRVO is under way.

Omar study – steroids reduced injection number, CRT but not VA in refractory CMO.

Generally, **data suggests that early response was a good predictor of longer-term behaviour** and a subsequent PRN protocol helps maintain long term vision.

5.3.3.7 Management of RVO

Management includes identifying at-risk patients and managing their ocular and systemic risk factors, to prevent RVO. **Involvement of a primary care physician is important, as RVO is a predictor of cardiovascular events (stroke, cardiac, and thromboembolic events) and for recurrent RVO in the fellow eye.**

Monitoring is important as 25% of CRVO patients will develop neovascularization.

Treatment is targeted at causes and sequelae of RVO. The aim is to:

- Treat all systemic and ocular risk factors.

- Improve or stabilize visual function.

- Detect and treat sight-threatening neovascular complications and macular oedema.

Several studies have shown safety and efficacy of IVT, with visual and anatomical benefits in comparison to laser or sham injections. Outcomes vary, with non-ischaemic patients achieving better results than ischaemic RVO patients.

Combination therapy with intravitreal sustained-release dexamethasone and an anti-VEGF agent is an emerging treatment to improve visual acuity and prolong injection intervals.

5.3.3.8 Treatment of Macular Oedema

Several RCTs support use of IVT (anti-VEGF and corticosteroids) for macular oedema in CRVO and BRVO, with no difference in outcomes with different agents. However, risks associated with steroids (cataract, high IOP) make anti-VEGF the preferred initial therapy.

First-line management – Anti-VEGF (Ranibizumab, aflibercept or Bevacizumab) **Standard treatment for MO in RVO and reduces VEGF drive for neovascularization.**
Second-line treatment – switch IVT to aflibercept if other agents used initially. *(Partially or non-responsive RVO, showed significant and sustained anatomical improvement when switched to Aflibercept).* **Switch to corticosteroids** if initial response sub-optimal
Third-line treatment – adjunct therapy (steroid + Anti-VEGF). A combination regime is useful, if long-term IVT is difficult or response is not sustained. Anti-VEGFs provides immediate results, while Dexa-implant sustains the response long term.
Fourth-line treatment – focal laser therapy in isolation or conjunction with IVT in BRVO. **50–75 shots × 100 um spot × 10 ms pulse × 100–200 mw power × Mainster focal lens.**

5.3.3.9 Laser Therapy in RVO

Two laser treatment strategies are **grid/focal and scatter PRP**.

- **GRID laser** – aims to reduce CMO or exudates and stabilize vision.

- **PRP** aims to reduce VEGF drive, by ablating peripheral ischaemic retina and reduce risk of neovascularization.

5.3.3.10 Laser Treatment for Macular Oedema

BVOS study – established benefit of FLT in perfused BRVO with MO with good outcomes.

CVOS study – did not show any value of focal or grid laser for CRVO-related MO. Treatment led to anatomic and angiographic improvement but no visual improvements.

However, CVOS used laser monotherapy as a treatment modality, where the presence of excessive fluid with severe MO was likely to make laser therapy ineffective. With the advent of new IVT and new lasers, it would be reasonable to explore laser therapy in conjunction with IVT. Once the CRT has been reduced by IVT, laser treatment may achieve a more sustained visual improvement, permanent resolution of MO, and reduce frequency of IVT.

5.3.3.11 When Is Laser Used in RVO-related Macular Oedema?

Anti-VEGF therapy is preferred due to better visual outcomes in BRVO. FLT may be considered if IVT is contraindicated or not suitable.

- Anxious patients who refuse IVT, needle phobia.

- Elderly patients, who cannot cope with recurrent injections, socio-economic reasons, lack of support to attend frequently.

- Medically unwell patients, where IVT may be unsuitable, or contraindicated.

- Presence of retinal exudates. IVT reduces retinal fluid, but not exudates.

Current concepts do not advocate the use of FLT in CRVO patients, but combination therapy and subthreshold laser treatment may prove useful in such cases.

5.3.4 Laser Treatment for Neovascularization

PRP is established treatment for ischaemic CRVO with anterior or posterior segment neovascularization (CVOS recommendation). The development of ocular NV usually occurs

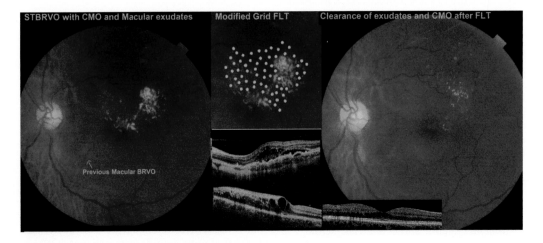

Figure 5.42 FLT for BRVO with exudates.

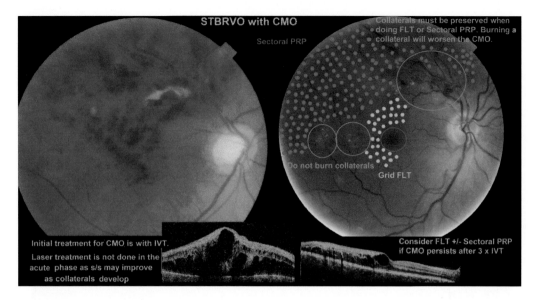

Figure 5.43 FLT in BRVO.

within 3 months of CRVO. Treatment aimed to prevent NV development should therefore be initiated early.

PRP should be early, aggressive, and completed in the shortest time possible.

IVT (anti-VEGF) can be used in ischaemic patients to reduce VEGF drive and prevent, delay, or reduce severity of neovascularization. IVT may buy time to complete PRP in elderly, medically unfit patients with vitreous haemorrhage or poor co-operation.

5.3.4.1 Laser Photocoagulation

CRVO	Urgent, aggressive PRP, completed within 1–2 weeks. Aim for 2500–3000 burns/session, repeat in 2–3 days, total of 5000–6000 burns in 2–3 sessions. PRP does not improve vision, but stabilizes RVO, reducing risk of progression and development of neovascular glaucoma.
HRVO	Sectoral PRP – target ischaemic quadrant (superior/inferior retina). Aim for 1500–2000 burns, to be completed in one session.
BRVO	Anterior segment neovascularization is rare but retinal NV can occur. Sectoral PRP, in the affected quadrant, to regress NV and reduce risk of vitreous haemorrhage. Aim for 1200–1500 burns, completed in one session. Watch out for and spare retinal collaterals to prevent worsening of MO.

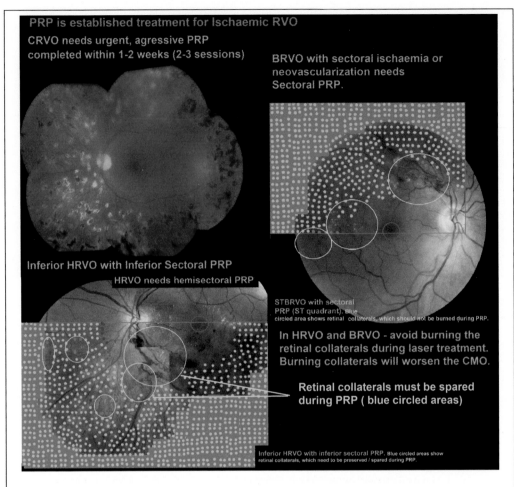

Figure 5.44 PRP in ischaemic RVO.

Prophylactic PRP in Presence of Clinical or Angiographic Features of Ischaemia
- *Although CVOS did not confirm benefit of prophylactic PRP in preventing NVG in CRVO, it was based on angiographic evidence of ischaemia, which, as discussed previously, can be subjective, variable, difficult to assess, and underestimated by FFA. More recent studies using UWFA and ERG-verified peripheral ischaemia suggest* **early PRP treatment is superior to standard treatment to prevent neovascular complications**.
- **Mild CRVO** with good VA and retinal perfusion, resolve spontaneously, and can be watched safely.
- **Moderate CRVO** – with modest visual loss and some ischaemia need regular monitoring and PRP at the earliest evidence of neovascularization.
- **Severe CRVO** – with poor vision (<6/60), RAPD, signs of ischaemia (CWS, extensive areas of non-perfusion), **has a high risk of rubeosis, and it is reasonable to consider prophylactic PRP,** to prevent anterior segment NV and development of painful blind eye.

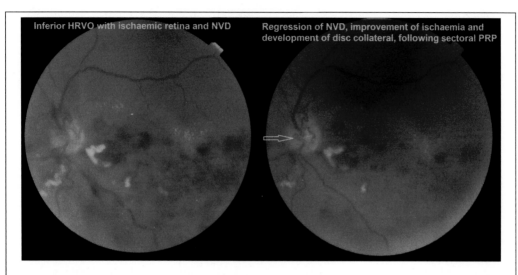

Inferior HRVO with ischaemic retina and NVD

Regression of NVD, improvement of ischaemia and development of disc collateral, following sectoral PRP

Figure 5.45 HRVO with NVD regression after PRP.

5.3.4.2 Outcomes in RVO

Location, severity of occlusion, and extent of ischaemia predict visual outcomes in RVO. Responses are variable and defining this is crucial to tailoring a patient-centric treatment regimen. Following three loading doses of anti-VEGF, the response can be categorized into:

- **Early/good responders** – CRT <250 um, patients do well long term (T&E or PRN).

- **Partial or non-responders** – CRT >250 um, further categorized as

  - Patients with <1% reduction in MO – non-responders

  - Patients with 10% reduction in MO – partial responders. Reload ×3, if responds, then T&E, if no/poor response – consider switch.

  - Non-responders may be offered three treatment options:

    - Switch to aflibercept.

    - Switch to dexamethasone implants

    - Steroid + anti-VEGF combination (synergic combination)

Poor responders (persistent fluid at 3 months) generally had worse outcomes at 6 and 12 months, with less visual gain, persistent fluid, and needing more injections. It is prudent to consider early therapy switch to prevent chronicity and achieve better long-term outcomes. **A 3-month OCT gives a reasonable indication to continuing treatment regimen or considering a switch to an alternate treatment modality.**

Final VA after resolution was better than 6/30 in only 12% of ischaemic CRVO patients compared with 83% in non-ischaemic patients. An estimated 30% of non-ischaemic cases tend to convert to ischaemic within 3 years, and the majority of eyes initially classified as indeterminate were non-perfused. Long-term treatment and follow-up is essential, until patients have been stable for more than a year.

SUGGESTED READING

1. Clinicaltrial.gov – all clinical trials in retinal vascular diseases

2. The DRS research Group. PRP treatment of PDR. Report no 8. *Ophthal.* 1981;88:583–600.

3. ETDRS Research Group. Techniques for scatter and local photocoagulation treatment of DR: report no. 2, 3, 9. *Int Ophthalmol Clin.* 1987;27(4):254–264.

4. Majcher, C. et al. A review of MPL photocoagulation. *Rev of Optometry.* 2011; Nov 10–17 (retinaguide pdf).

5. Wells, J.A. et al. Aflibercept, bevacizumab or ranibizumab for DME. *N Engl J Med.* 2015;372:1193–1203.

6. Martin, D.R. Treatment choice for DME. *N Engl J Med.* 2015. Feb 18;371(13):1260–1261. doi: 10.1056/NEJMe1500351. Epub 2015 Feb 18.

7. Bakri, S.J. et al. Evidence based guidelines for management of DME. *J VR disease.* 2019;3:145–152.

8. Bressler, S.B. et al. Photocoagulation vs ranibizumab for PDR: should baseline characteristics affect choice of treatment? *Retina.* 2019;39:1646–1654.

9. Beaulieu, W.T et al. PRP vs ranibizumab for PDR: patient centred outcomes. *Am J Ophth .* 2016;170:206–213.

10. Tah, V. et al. Anti-VEGF therapy and the retina: An update. *J Ophthal.* 2015;627674. doi: 10.1155/2015/627674. Epub 2015 Aug 31.

11. Ehlers, J.P. et al. Automated quantitative characterization of retinal vascular leakage and mA in UWFA. *BJO.* 2017;101:696–699.

12. Tan, C.S. et al. Measuring precise area of peripheral retinal non-perfusion using UWFA. *BJO.* 2016;100:235–239.

13. Vemala, R. et al. Qualitative and quantitative OCT response of diffuse MO to macular laser photocoagulation. Published online 2011 Apr 15. doi: 10.1038/eye.2011.84 PMID: 21494279.

14. Romero-Aroca, P. et al. NPDR and DME progression after phacoemulsication: prospective study. *J Cataract Refract Surg.* 2006;32(9):1438–1444.

15. Elman, M.J. et al. Intravitreal ranibizumab for DME with prompt versus deferred laser treatment: 5-year results. *Ophthalmology.* 2015;122(2):375–381.

16. Mehta, H. et al. Combination of anti-VEGFand laser therapy for DME: a review. *Clin Experiment Ophthalmol.* 2016;44(4):335–339.

17. El Annan, J. et al. Current management of vitreous haemorrhage due to PDR. *Int Ophth Clin.* 2014;54(2):141–153.

18. Salam, A. et al. Treatment of PDR with anti-VEGF agents. *Acta Ophthalmol.* 2011;89(5):405–411

19. Osaadon, P. et al. A review of anti-VEGF agents for PDR. *Eye (Lond).* 2014;28(5):510–520.

20. Neubauer, A.S. et al. Laser treatment in DR. *Ophthalmologica.* 2007;221(2):95–102.

21. Lee, C.M. et al. Modified grid laser for diffuse DME. Long-term visual results. *Ophthalm.* 1991;98(10):1594–1602.

22. Stefánsson, E. The therapeutic effects of retinal laser treatment and vitrectomy. A theory based on oxygen and vascular physiology. *Acta Ophthalmol Scand.* 2001;79(5):435–440.

23. Navarro, A. et al. Vitrectomy may prevent occurrence of DME. *Acta Ophthalmol.* 2010;88:483–485.

24. Gandorfer, A. et al. DME resolution after surgical removal of posterior hyaloid and ILM. *Retina.* 2000;20:126–133.

25. Stolba, U. et al. Vitrectomy for persistent diffuse DME. *Am J Ophthalmol.* 2005;140:295–301.

26. Antonetti, D.A. Diabetic retinopathy. *N Engl J Med.* 2012;366(13):1227–1239.

27. Srivastav, K. et al. OCT biomarkers as functional outcome predictors in DME treated with dexa-implant. *Ophthalmology.* 2018;125:267–275.

28. Oliver, S.C.N. et al. Peripheral vessel leakage (PVL): A new angiographic finding in DR identified with UWFA. *Sem Ophthalmol.* 2010; 25:27–33.

29. Hayreh, S.S. et al. Differentiation of ischaemic from non-ischaemic CRVO during the early acute phase. *Graefe's Arch Clin Exp Ophthal.* 1999; 228:201–217.

30. Spaide, R.F. Peripheral areas of nonperfusion in treated CRVO as imaged by UWFA. *Retina.* 2011;31:829–837.

31. CVOS group. Evaluation of grid pattern photocoagulation for MO in CRVO. *Ophthalmology.* 1995;102:1425–1433.

32. BVOS Group. Argon laser photocoagulation for MO in BRVO. *Am J Ophth.* 1984;98:271–282.

33. Larson, J. et al. Photopic 30 Hz flicker ERG as a predictor for rubeosis in CRVO. *BJO*. 2001;85(6):683–685.

34. Di Capua, M. et al. Cardiovascular risk factors and outcomes in RVO. *J Thromb Thrombolysis*. 2010;30:16–22.

35. Singer, M. et al. Areas of peripheral non-perfusion and treatment response in RVO. *Retina*. 2014;34:1736–1742.

36. Campochiaro, P.A. et al. Scatter photocoagulation does not reduce macular edema or treatment burden in RVO: The Relate trial. *Ophthalmology*. 2015 Jul; 122(7):1426–1437.

37. BVOS Group. Argon laser scatter photocoagulation for prevention of neovascularization and vitreous hemorrhage in BRVO. A randomized clinical trial. *Arch Ophthalmol*. 1986; 104:34–41.

38. Rehak, M. et al. Early peripheral laser photocoagulation on nonperfused retina improves vision in patients with CRVO. *Graefes Arch Clin Exp Ophthalmol*. 2014; 252:745–752.

Acknowledgement of Images Borrowed

Section 2		
1	Figure 2.1	**YAG Laser machine – Courtesy of Lumenis** – *courtesy of Lumenis*
2	Figure 2.34	**YAG posterior synechiolysis** (modification of original image) – *Courtesy of Maria Papadoupoulou, Feb 2017; Ácta Ophthalmologica 95(7)*
3	Figure 2.40	**CMO with vitreous wick syndrome** – *Courtesy of Retina Gallery; cme_roen_08281514_copy.jpg, Album name: scohen125 / CME*
4	Figure 2.45	**Subhyaloid and preretinal haemorrhage** – *Courtesy of Retina Gallery* *1. PDR – Preretinal Hemorrhage – may2012; James L. Perron, C.R.A.* *2. rupturedma.png; Album name: scohen125 / Arterial Macroaneurysm* *3. scherfFPWA1r~0.jpg; Album name: Macroaneurysm/ january2013; Marissa Scherf* *4. VH_WITH_PDR~0.jpg; PDR Subhyaloid Hemorrhage: Southwest Retina*
5	Figure 2.46	**Subhyaloid haemorrhage treated with YAG hyaloidotomy** – *Courtesy of Retina Gallery; scherfFPWA1r~0.jpg; / Macroaneurysm/ january2013; Marissa Scherf*
Section 3		
6	Figure 3.7	**YAG LPI -1** – *Courtesy of Retina Gallery; 145_004.JPG; Album name:/ PI: Mayo Clinic Jacksonville, Florida, Jul 12, 2014*
7	Figure 3.8	**LPI with iris haemorrhage and hyphema** – *Courtesy of Retina Gallery 24050_006_PNG. jpg; Mayo Clinic Jacksonville, Florida*
8	**Figure 3.15**	**SLT vs ALT** – *Digital drawing of original image, L. Jay Katz, MD, Philadelphia*
Section 4		
9	Figure 4.1 Figure 4.2 Figure 4.3 Figure 4.4 Figure 4.5 Figure 4.6	**Parts of Laser – PASCAL** **PASCAL laser** **PASCAL home page and menu page** **Menu screen – posterior segment display page 2** **Variety of patterns for PRP and Retinopexy-1 Patterns for FLT**	*Courtesy of Iridex*
10	Figure 4.12	**FFA in PRP;** *Courtesy of Retina gallery pdr_erfr_1013_28.jpg; scohen125 / PDR – Non-perfusion and NVD and NVE*
11	Figure 4.13	**FFA in PRP-2** – *Courtesy of Retina Gallery* *PDR_kaco_102918_21.jpg, Album name: scohen125 / Severe PDR with preretinal fibrosis* *pdr_alebek_041819_15.jpg; Album name: scohen125 / Moderate PDR*
12	Figure 4.16	**FFA in PRP-3;** *Courtesy of Retina Gallery* *pdr_erfr_1013_28.jpg; Album name: scohen125 / PDR – Non-perfusion and NVD and NVE*
13	Figure 4.23	*1. PDR with NVD, NVE and preretinal haemorrhage (1); Courtesy of Retina gallery* *James L Perron, CRA* *2. Courtesy of Retina gallery 49823_002.JPG; Macular Pre-Retinal Haemorrhage, Mayo Clinic, Florida*
14	4.29	**Fibrosed NVD and NVE with retinal distortion** – *Courtesy of Retina Gallery 168663_001.JPG Albumi nimi:/ PDR Võtmesõnad:/ august2014; Carolina Eye Associates*
15	Figure 4.46	**STBRVO with peripheral ischaemia** – *Courtesy of Retina Gallery* *VANDERLAANR12.jpg; Album name: Peripheral Ischemia:: Kathy Karsten, COT. Retina Specialists of Michigan*
16	Figure 4.95	**Nasal exudates treated with FLT** – *Courtesy of Retina Gallery; 51171_010.JPG; Album name: DR:: Mayo Clinic Jacksonville, Florida*
17	Figure 4.104	**EPM menu page** – *Courtesy of Iridex*
18	Figure 4.105	**Clearance of exudates after FLT** – *Courtesy of Retina Gallery; 51354_003.JPG, Album name: DR with Scattered Haemorrhages::Mayo Clinic Jacksonville, Florida*
19	Figures 4.96, 4.107 & 4.108 Figure 5.12	**Bilateral severe exudative maculopathy** – *Courtesy of Retina gallery; 50204_003.JPG Album name: BDR, Mayo Clinic Jacksonville, Florida* *50204_011.JPG Album name: BDR, Mayo Clinic Jacksonville, Florida*
20	4.112	**FTMH, Macular pucker** – *Courtesy of Retina Gallery* *1. SymphonyWeb163709_1.jpg; Album name:/ Macular Hole* *2. VMT-machole-nabr-031218-04_copy.jpg; Album name: scohen125* *3. machole_PPV_IOL_051918_caku_09.jpg; Album name: scohen125 / Macular Hole* *4. 430_001.JPG, Macular Pucker; Album name: Võtmesõnad: september2014:: Mayo Clinic Jacksonville, Florida* *5. puckerspontpeeled_frva03.png; Album name: scohen125 / Macular Pucker – Spontaneously Partially Peeled*
21	Figure 4.116	**Heavy FLT with macular scar** – *Courtesy of Retina Gallery; macularlaser-dm-leer_28129. png; Album name: scohen125 / Macular Laser Scars – DR*

22	Figure 4.129	**RAM with haemorrhage-1** – *Courtesy of Retina Gallery, arrows.jpg and mavisit1_faca09.jpg; Album name: scohen125 / Arterial Macroaneurysm*
23	Figure 4.134	**RAM with leak** – *Courtesy of Retina Gallery; ANDERSON_RICHARD_5B0035D; album name – Coats' disease*
24	Figure 4.141	**CSCR-1** – *Courtesy Retina gallery; csrsmokestack_blma12.jpg Album name: scohen125 / Acute CSCR – Classic Smokestack*
25	Figure 4.142	**CSCR with OCT changes** – *Courtesy of Retina Gallery; csr_60031_281129.jpg, Album name: scohen125 / CSR – PED and Serous RD*
26	Figure 4.145	**IJFT** – *Courtesy of Retina Gallery – mactelnelupreheme2007.jpg Album name: scohen125 / Juxtafoveal Telangiectasia*
27	Figure 4.147	**Type 2 IJFT** – *Courtesy of Retina Gallery – ijft_blti_28329.jpg; Album name: scohen125 / Juxta foveal Telangiectasis – Good VA + Crystals*
28	Figure 4.148	**Type 2 IJFT-1** – *Courtesy of Retina Gallery.* 1. *ijft_knud02.png, Album name: scohen125 / Juxta foveal Telangiectasis – Group 2a – MacTel* 2. *jft5_keha14.png, Album name: scohen125 / Juxta foveal Telangiectasis – Stage 5 Spectralis*
29	Figure 4.149 Figure 4.152	**Type 3 IJFT** – *Courtesy of Retina Gallery type3IJFT_arwh_120613_21.jpg Album name: scohen125 / Obliterative – Type 3 Juxtafoveal Telangiectasis*
30	Figure 4.153	**Retinal degeneration** – *Lattice degeneration and WWOP- Courtesy of Optos; Retinoschisis – Courtesy of Retina Gallery, rs_mamc_051616_03.jpg Album:scohen125 / Bullous Retinoschisis – Superior*
31	Figure 4.157	**Laser retinopexy for horseshoe retinal tear** – *Courtesy of Retina Gallery – 43536_001.JPG; Album name:/ Retinal Tears, Mayo Clinic Jacksonville*
32	Figure 4.158	**Laser retinopexy is not appropriate for these conditions** – *Courtesy of Retina Gallery* 1. *Giantdialysisrd_masc07.jpg; Album name: scohen125 / Dialysis* 2. *28047_006.PNG; Album name: Retinal Tears, Mayo Clinic* 3. *29990_001.JPG; Album name: Retinal Tears, Mayo Clinic* 4. *39823_014.JPG; Album name: Retinal Tears, Mayo Clinic, Jacksonville*
33	Figure 4.159	**Retinal tears with Retinal detachment** – *Courtesy of Retina Gallery* 1. *50389_001.JPG, Album name: RD – with retinal tear: Mayo Clinic Jacksonville, Florida* 2. *50507_001.JPG; Album name: Horseshoe Tear with RD*
34	Figure 4.161	**Retinopexy menu page** – *Courtesy of Iridex*
35	Figure 4.162	**Laser retinopexy for operculated hole with localised RD** – *Courtesy of Retina Gallery – subclinicalRD_jojen_021720_01.jpg Album name:scohen125*
36	Figure 4.163	**Extremely peripheral tear** – *Courtesy of Retina Gallery, Tear_CRT_laser_jebru.jpg; Album name: scohen125 / Lasered retinal tear with cystic retinal tuft*
37	Figure 4.164	**Retinopexy with lattice degeneration** – *Courtesy of Optos*
Section 5		
38	Figure 5.9	**Montage of PDR** – *Courtesy of Retina Gallery* 1. *PDR_kaco 102918_06.JPG; Album name: scohen125 / PDR with preretinal fibrosis* 2. *49295_007.JPG; Album name: Rubeosis Iridis, Mayo Clinic Jacksonville, Florida* 3. *PDR.jpg; Album name: Juvenile Onset Diabetic – PDR with NVE and NVD Võtmesõnad: july2012:: James L. Perron, C.R.A.*
39	Figure 5.10	**Montage of end stage PDR** – *Courtesy of Retina Gallery* 1. *RD_with_Macular_Hole_OD.jpg; Album name: Diabetic Pre-retinal Fibrosis: Goiania Eye Institute* 2. *50921_002.JPG; Album name: Proliferative Diabetic Retinopathy::Mayo Clinic Jacksonville, Florida* 3. *49772_004~0.JPG; Album name: Prominent Posterior Hyaloid with BDR::Mayo Clinic Jacksonville, Florida* 4. *444_001.JPG; Vitreo-Traction due to DR::Mayo Clinic Jacksonville, Florida* 5. *heavy_PRP_labro_01.png; Album name:scohen125 / Heavy PRP for PDR and TRD – 1981 (PRP) Scarring* 6. *168663_001.JPG; Album name: PDR:: Carolina Eye* 7. *pdrvhos_stpo_28529.png; Album name:scohen125 / Vitreous Haemorrhage*

Index

Note: Page numbers in *italics* indicate figures on the corresponding pages.